PRAISE FOR

EMBRACE YOGA'S ROOTS

"I can't think of anyone more suited to lead the way to embrace yoga's roots than Susanna. This book should be required reading in yoga teacher trainings across the world."

—**RACHEL BRATHEN**, AUTHOR OF *YOGA GIRL*

"A must have for any teacher or practitioner of yoga wishing to embrace its lineage."

—**KATHRYN BUDIG,** FOUNDER OF AIM TRUE

"Susanna Barkataki's words are vital medicine for yoga today. Study, absorb and share this with your community—watch the lines of communication open and expand."

—**ELENA BROWER,** BESTSELLING AUTHOR OF *PRACTICE YOU AND ART OF ATTENTION*

"You must read this book."

—**AMBER KARNES,** FOUNDER, BODY POSITIVE YOGA

"*Embrace Yoga's Roots* should become a curricular text in all yoga teacher training programs and essential reading for anyone wanting to understand the

effects of cultural appropriation, race and white supremacy. We have an opportunity to change the tide and Susanna Barkataki is uniquely qualified to act as our guide."

—**DONNA FARHI,** AUTHOR OF *YOGA MIND, BODY AND SPIRIT: A RETURN TO WHOLENESS*

"*Embrace Yoga's Roots* is a crucial addition to every yoga practitioner's bookshelf."

—**JESSAMYN STANLEY,** AUTHOR OF *EVERY BODY YOGA*, FOUNDER OF THE UNDERBELLY YOGA

"Susanna Barkataki is a bold, fearless leader who is leading the charge in decolonizing yoga."

—**JESAL PARIKH,** YOGA IS DEAD CO-FOUNDER, YOGAWALLA

"Required reading for anyone who teaches yoga, works as a healer or is interested in equity and equality on the mat."

—**DIANNE BONDY,** FOUNDER OF YOGA FOR ALL YOGA TEACHER TRAINING 200/300/500

"Her words are like water washing away the confusion around cultural appropriation with clear thinking, *viveka*, allowing us to move into a new chapter in yoga's ancient history—one that harkens back to a tradition which has always been equitable, inclusive and accessible at its heart."

—JIVANA HEYMAN,
ACCESSIBLE YOGA FOUNDER
AND DIRECTOR

"Susanna's commitment to the themes of roots and healing is needed for our world to be in equanimity, unity and connection!"

—HEMALAYAA BEHL,
YOGINI, TRANSFORMATIONAL
FACILITATOR, EMBODY
LEADERSHIP COACH

"This is it. The long-overdue conversation that has been swept under the rug year after year. It's a call to action for the yoga community as a whole. Teachers, students, practitioners—this book is for you. It's for all of us."

—NADIA CARRIERE,
FOUNDER OF THE UNIVERSAL
SCHOOL OF YOGA

"She beautifully guides us through discourse, doable steps, and refined tools; all designed to aid readers in building an authentic yoga practice."

—MAYA BREUER,
E-RYT 500 EMERITUS TRUSTEE,
KRIPALU CENTER FOR YOGA
AND HEALTH

"*Embrace Yoga's Roots* gives us a roadmap back to the heart of a practice meant to be about liberation for all beings, not just individual wellbeing."

—HALA KHOURI, M.A., SEP,
CO-FOUNDER OFF THE MAT,
INTO THE WORLD

"Susanna Barkataki gently illuminates a path back from highly processed modern yoga to its nutritive, medicinal root—liberation. The world needs this book now more than ever!"

—LAKSHMI NAIR,
SATYA YOGA COOPERATIVE

"Barkataki has given us a practical guidebook to help deepen our understanding of yoga's rich history so as to preserve the integrity of its future growth. I highly recommend this book."

—SEANE CORN,
CO-FOUNDER, OFF THE MAT,
INTO THE WORLD, AUTHOR OF
REVOLUTION OF THE HEART

"Susanna has created a gift to our yoga community that should be a part of all yoga teacher trainings and on the shelf of all teachers and practitioners."

—KELLEY PALMER,
SOLUTION ARCHITECT, MAMA,
YOGI, WRITER, ADVOCATE

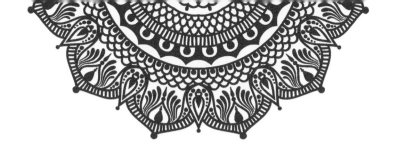

EMBRACE

COURAGEOUS WAYS TO

YOGA'S

DEEPEN YOUR YOGA PRACTICE

ROOTS

SUSANNA BARKATAKI

Ignite Yoga and Wellness Institute
P.O. Box 536074
Orlando, Florida 32803

www.ignitebewell.com

Publisher's Cataloging-In-Publication Data
(Prepared by The Donohue Group, Inc.)

Names: Barkataki, Susanna, author.
Title: Embrace yoga's roots : courageous ways to deepen your practice / Susanna Barkataki.
Description: Orlando, Florida : Ignite Yoga and Wellness Institute, [2020] | Includes bibliographical references and index.
Identifiers: ISBN 9781734318111 (black and white) | ISBN 9781734318104 (color) | ISBN 9781734318128 (ebook)
Subjects: LCSH: Yoga--History. | Yoga--Social aspects. | Philosophy, Asian. | Social justice. | Cultural appropriation. | Mind and body. | BISAC: HEALTH & FITNESS / Yoga.
Classification: LCC BL1238.52 .B37 2020 (print) | LCC BL1238.52 (ebook) | DDC 181.45--dc23

Paperback ISBN: 978-1-7343181-1-1
eBook ISBN: 978-1-7343181-2-8

Printed in the United States of America

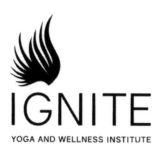

WELCOME TO
EMBRACE YOGA'S ROOTS: COURAGEOUS WAYS TO DEEPEN YOUR PRACTICE

If you would like to jumpstart your exploration of the traditions of yoga and want to immediately integrate that knowledge into your practice while preparing for the deeper lessons presented in this book, Susanna has created a complementary video masterclass to accompany this book on how to start and end your yoga class confidently while embracing yoga's roots.

Extend your learning and get support for your journey to bring the yoga tradition alive in your practice and honor its roots now.

www.namastemasterclass.com

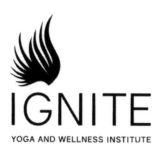

IGNITE

YOGA AND WELLNESS INSTITUTE

CONTENTS

IV
REFLECTION

VII
HOW TO CONTINUE THIS WORK

Aum.

Asato ma sad-gamaya;

tamaso ma jyotir-gamaya;

mrtyor-ma amrutam gamaya.

Aum.

Shanti, shanti, shanti.

Aum.

Lead me from unreal to real;

lead me from darkness to light;

lead me from death to immortality.

Aum.

Peace, peace, peace.

— Brihadaranyaka Upanishad 1.3.28

A DEDICATION AND INVOCATION TO THIS PRACTICE

INVOCATION

Om Shanti, Shanti, Shanti

Let us embrace yoga's roots and honor our teachers together.

I honor my teachers. I honor your teachers.

I embrace all the elements, earth, water, fire, air and space.
I embrace the land and the sky and all of creation.

I honor the yogis back through time and space.
I honor my colleagues, friends, co-conspirators on this path.

I honor the students, known and unknown,
whose lives will be touched by this work.

May we embrace the roots of yoga
so the tree of vast yogic wisdom can abundantly flourish.

Welcome to this inquiry and practice.

May it benefit you, may it preserve and uplift the practice and path of
yoga now and for generations to come. May it benefit all beings.

Om Shanti, Shanti, Shanti

FOREWORD

BY SONALI FISKE

I had only practiced yoga in-studio, just once in my life. In November of 2014 to be exact.

Opening the door to the studio, I was met with a whiff of sandalwood incense. Hindu deities were carefully arranged on a long back shelf, bright red Sanskrit murals were gracing the walls, and a carousel of yoga magazines were for sale. An *Om* symbol drew you into the back room, where folks were scoping out the most optimal spot on the ground.

I sat down toward the back end of the room, and slowly surveyed the space. In that freeze-frame moment, I was hyper aware that yoga had a look. And that look was also wholly white. I was the sole person of color in that space. A damp sweat started developing on my upper lip. My stomach was beginning to slow churn. And I was shallow breathing too. My body knew it didn't belong there.

Looking back now, I know it was a revelation. That small space was a microcosm for the everyday real-world trauma black and brown folks carry in their bodies due to white dominance.

But how did we get here? How was I, a person of South Asian descent, practicing a discipline as a "guest" when I belong to the culture from which it stemmed?

This isn't a foray into existentialism, but it leads into exactly why Susanna's work and this book is so necessary—she requires you to self-inquire and deepen every question, so that you can begin to do less harm to folks of color, as you practice yoga.

Susanna's earnest connection to her ancestral lineage, rooted in India, is how she stays power-sourced for this work. She's the real deal. She requires a certain squirming in your seat, or in this case, on your yoga mat, as a throughway to doing better.

I love Susanna's belief in the unifying power of yoga. But not at the expense of bypassing the racism, exclusion and co-option that is so blatant to her. As she says: "saying '*but we are all one*' denies the systemic injustice, harm and pain many have experienced because it makes you uncomfortable."

She is fiercely driven to ensuring folks of color are prioritized and made to feel safe and welcomed in yoga spaces. Because she is painfully familiar with what exclusion feels like to her and the coaches and practitioners of color when she said: "Brown people are not props or photo ops for your good feelings."

She believes that yoga is a consistent checking-in with yourself, being willing to ask: "Is what I am doing creating more separation or more unity?"

Because if your yoga is causing harm and alienating folks of color, it doesn't count.

If you are grabbing fragmented pieces of yoga culture without any historical context or any regard for the origins of it, you are causing harm.

If you have no regard for who else is in the room, or more accurately, you have no regard for who else *isn't* in the room, you are causing harm.

If you are blasé about the clear power dynamics at play—how folks of a dominant culture cherry-pick incomplete parts of a culture from a people who have been systemically oppressed by that dominant culture—you are causing harm.

If your yoga practice is taken and with force—that is, there's no mutual exchange or agreement, or you have no deeper understanding of its lineage or history—you are causing harm.

If you've made it this far, keep going. Do the work. Do the book. Take your time with the reflection questions Susanna has carefully crafted for you to dive deeper into yourself.

Susanna's book is a firm commitment to doing better. But she will be the first to tell you that this book is only the gateway to doing and being better. It is merely the launch point.

Because doing this book is not restorative justice. Because while you're receiving your education through *Embrace Yoga's Roots*, as you are unlearning the harm, as you journal and self-reflect, on the flip side of this, people of marginalized identities are being re-traumatized in a yoga studio, online or in their neighborhood every day. Unfortunately, there's no stop sign on appropriation.

Every journey into unlearning, doing better, restorative healing and reparation, has a beginning. And you begin today.

GLOBAL EMPATHY, THE SPARK THAT BRINGS THIS WORK ALIVE

I AM SITTING IN MY USUAL SPOT ON MY SQUISHY BROWN SOFA, ON UN-ceded Seminole land, tropical heat rising from the lush greenery outside, my sweet puppy Harmony is curled up in the corner, sleeping. A cup of home-blended spiced *chai* is steaming on the table. Behind me on the wall, next to a sparkling red *diya*, candle, softly flickering as I write, reflecting off the *puja*, an altar holds space across time and location. An image of Mt. Kailash, Shiva's sacred abode, towers above my shoulders reminding me of the land, ancestors, future generations and the present moment are all alive in this moment.

I breathe in with anticipation, I breathe out with resolve.

You are present too. I see us here. Sitting on this comfy sofa, side by side. Together, we get to explore how to practice yoga with unity and respect in a world full of separation and appropriation.

As we talk we explore how you are similar to me in so many ways. And in other ways you are so different. I trust and know that when we explore like this, when we address separation, difference, uniqueness as well as similarity, we enable ourselves to move toward true unity.

This takes courage for both of us.

We are, at this moment perhaps more than ever, seeing how intercon-nected we all are.

Yoga brings us a message and practical step-by-step guide for personal, local and global connectedness. It also invites us into an increased capacity for universal empathy.

I invite you to travel with me on this journey that explores separation as we move through it as a key towards our global empathy, unity and oneness.

You see, to be colonized is to become a stranger in your own land and culture. As an Indian woman, this is often the feeling I get in many Westernized yoga spaces today.

I've been ignored, kicked out and uninvited to teach in yoga festivals and spaces, been looked up and down in yoga classes as if I didn't belong, had teachers dismiss me except to ask me how to pronounce Sanskrit words, and when I raised concerns about how a practice didn't sit well with me or folks in my family, been completely ignored or even mocked.

I've grieved the loss of the wisdom of my ancestors robbed from us by colonization, and once again taken and reduced to tips for getting a better "yoga [insert sexualized body part]."

I've shed tears of frustration at so many of us being shut out by yoga institutions in the West. I've written letters, called, spoken up, campaigned and cried, listened and laughed for over two decades.

This brings me here. There is so much work to do. I've desired for so long to have the deep practice I know and love from my family and teachers in the tradition be shared far and wide. I want nothing more than this practice that we cherish to be embraced and respected, taught in its fullness for us and for future generations. And I'm still here.

I'm here, despite the frustration, grief, desperation I've felt at times. I'm here because of the promise of liberation that this practice has offered me, you and so many. I hope to preserve it for future generations.

This aim takes you, it takes me, it takes an entire yoga community. It takes all of us. I continue to speak, to teach, to write to reconnect myself as well as to reconnect with you.

There are many different perspectives and experiences to bring to light in this exploration. Including your own.

I am writing as a culturally mixed, diasporic Indian living in the West, addressing Western readers. Please understand there may be some considerations beyond the scope of this book. Some of what I write will speak to Desis, Indians and Black Indigenous People of Color and some of what I write will speak to white folks. This is an invitation to global empathy. I hope there is ample nourishment here for us all within our unique perspectives as we engage with yoga for unity and liberation for all.

This book and exploration will invite you to explore your own depths and heights. It will invite you to feel deeply.

At times, this exploration may feel uncomfortable. It has for me writing it. At times, it may feel incredibly joyful and inspiring. Sometimes it may feel messy. You may have more questions than answers. At times, you may leap up with an Ah-ha! of great understanding. Sometimes this exploration may be uncomfortable or isolating. You may feel anger, denial or a desire to defend. You may feel triggered—and I invite you to remember you are in the right place and keep reading. My hope is that you will sit with the range of emotions as you delve into this book.

I am here with you, for it all. Holding your hand and sitting by your side on this journey. I am a full and complex being. At times, I may feel like a kind friend, and other times a provocative devil's advocate or challenging coach. Know that I show up with the energy of connection. I write with the spirit of yoga, of unity and love, inviting *satya*, truth and *ahimsa*, non-harm, into our yogic life. We are here together to speak truth and invite inquiry.

Together, we will embark on this exploration through this book and in our lives. We will explore a process for embracing rather than diluting yoga. This book follows an arc. We begin and examine what separates us, then reflect on our parts, learn how to take action for equity, and finally move toward liberation together. Please continue through the entire journey, even if at times you feel like giving up. Just like in yoga class, listen, practice and stay with me to the end.

We have some inspiring work to do! We will examine yoga as a science of personal liberation and social justice.

The anchor for us both is the trust in this practice of yoga that carries us through. The practice that invites us into inner empowerment and outer transformation and uplift.

I can't wait to start exploring the yogic traditions of the past, bringing them alive today, and preserving them for the future. Thank you for being a part of this movement to embrace and not appropriate yoga.

With great passion, love and a deep bow,

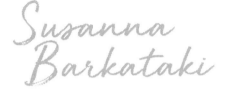

I
INTRODUCTION

"All revolutions are spiritual at the source."

—Vinoba Bhave

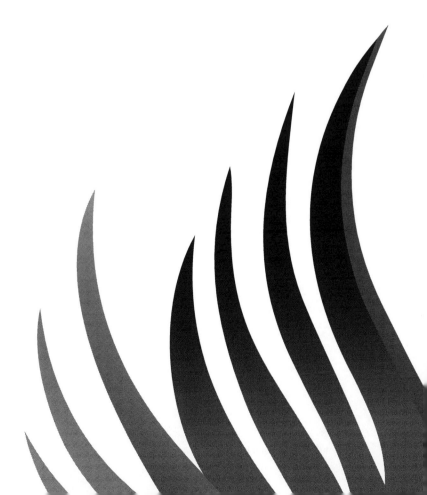

WHAT IS YOGA?

THERE HAVE BEEN SOME MISUNDERSTANDINGS AS TO WHAT YOGA IS IN the West today. The problem with these misunderstandings is they dilute yogic teachings to the point where yoga is barely recognizable at all.

Change is always happening, so why does this matter, you may ask?

At its root yoga is a practical, structured, scientific framework and embodiment practice that aims at curing our personal and social ills.

The *Yoga Sutras* of *Patanjali*, one of the seminal texts of yogic practice alongside the *Bhagavad Gita*, share 195 aphorisms that guide us to ways to practice yoga.

In the *Yoga Sutras*, it is said that *Patanjali* sought to organize the various practices of yoga that were shared by many different yogis. The *sutras* were told and then written during a cultural context where spiritual aspiration and practice was highly valued. This time was one where many renunciates were practicing to lessen human suffering and find liberation, under trees, by rivers and streams, in caves and on the outskirts of villages. The 195 *sutras* are guidelines to this practice of yoga.

At the very beginning of the *Yoga Sutras,* we learn that we will begin, now. Here in the present moment with a discussion of yoga.

The second *shloka* goes on to describe what yoga is and how to attain it.

1.2 YOGAŚ CITTA VRTTI NIRODHAH
(*The Yoga Sutras of Patanjali*, Translation and Commentary by Sri Swami Satchidananda. Integral Yoga Publications. 1978)

The Yoga Sūtras of Patañjali are 196 short aphorisms written by the sage Patañjali between 500 BCE and 400 CE in India.

Yoga is the calming of the fluctuations of the mind in order to find unity within. When we are able to calm our own mental talk and find a sense of ease, we begin to unite our small 's' self with our large 'S' Self. This unity comes by bringing mind, body and heart into harmony. Yoga is both the result of this practice and the mind training that brings us into the joy of being fully present in this very moment.

1.12 ABHYĀSA VAIRĀGYĀBHYĀM TANNIRODHAH

Through dedicated practice and an unattached heart, we enter into union with ourselves and experience our connection and unity with everything else. Through choosing to cultivate a practice of union with ourselves, we invite freedom and liberation again and again.

But there are so many obstacles to unity with ourselves and with others that exist for us today.

Our hearts may expand, numb or cry out with the immensity of challenges humankind faces today. We are grappling with so many challenges, from environmental destruction, to social inequity and spiritual harm such as relentless insomnia, anxiety and depression. As the earth's temperature rises and environmental impacts hit the world's most vulnerable, we also see suicide rates rise to alarming levels among our youngest and most vulnerable populations in the developed world.

There are many valiant efforts to address issues such as pollution, harm to animals, racism, sexism, classism, homophobia and other practices of separation and abuses of power. All of these are necessary. What yoga offers us is a pathway to know within ourselves the root cause of so many of these harms: separation.

Yoga provides a guided pathway of practice to live, experience, feel and act for unity now and into the future. It gives us a plan and pathway of action, in our own hearts, thoughts, bodies and actions. A pathway we can follow, step by step.

To save our planet will take great collaboration. We need to work across lines of difference, see no one as other, build and cooperate in ways we haven't yet anticipated.

Take a moment to zoom out in your mind's eye. Imagine yourself looking at Earth from space, this small, green-blue ball, that we all have as our mothership, our home; there might arise an inevitable feeling of humble insignificance, as well as a feeling of subtle connection with every other being on the planet. What are borders in the face of environmental destruction? Healthy and unhealthy air does not maintain citizenship status nor know racial divides. Clean water cares not for immigration laws.

Just as the view of our earth from space reminds us, yoga teaches us again and again the intimate truth of our ultimate interconnection. Connection with self and connection with one another. We are all interconnected.

When we mistake yoga for a workout routine, reduce it to physical fitness or even practice some of the deeper practices without an eye to the whole system of liberation it offers, we rob ourselves and each other of the potential of this practice.

However, the solution to this problem isn't hard.

Though we have made some mistakes and gotten confused in our practice of yoga in the West, the criteria for practicing yoga itself is quite simple.

Anything not leading toward unity is not yoga.

Yoga takes us right to complete connection. As *Krishna* reminds us in the *Bhagavad Gita*, "do every action you must do, but do not be attached to your actions' fruits." We don't even need to try to connect.

We are always already connected.

If our thought, speech or action is not bringing us right there, toward connection, it is not yoga.

After all, ultimately, yoga is *yuj*, union, unity. We will explore practical ways to bring this experience alive for ourselves, for others, for the yoga community in the West and for society.

And we have no time to waste as what hangs in the balance is the preciousness of each moment and a future that is possible with embracing the depth of yoga's true path of unity and liberation.

HOW TO USE THIS TEXT AND WHO THIS BOOK IS FOR

This text offers a deep dive into the problems that confront yoga today, along with several healing practices. It offers an arc of exploration that leads us toward justice, healing and equity as well as how we can embrace yoga's roots.

You can use this text by going right through: reading and inquiring as you do. Or, you can turn to specific sections when you have questions. You can also revisit sections after exploring new texts or taking more yoga training.

This book is for any person who practices, teaches or is curious about yoga.

Together we are developing empathy as we consider the relative ways we may differ in experiences as we move towards the shared aim of yoga as unity.

It doesn't matter how long you've been practicing or where. This process is for any student, devoted practitioner, teacher, studio owner, nonprofit or business owner who wants to understand cultural appropriation and properly embrace their practice.

It's for you, if you've ever been unsure, insecure or curious about how to practice yoga without causing harm. Even the best-intentioned can cause harm by taking yoga out of context or diluting the practice. Harm can also be caused when people aren't aware of the culture and traditions from which yoga comes, and unintentionally disrespect cultural elements of yoga.

For example, someone who is beginning to work with deities from the yoga pantheon may take a deity, such as *Ganesh*, the elephant-headed god, and place him on the floor or by the shoe rack in the studio. In Indian culture, one pays great respect to anything that represents divine energy and would never place a deity on the floor or by shoes. So even with good intentions, without knowledge, harm can be caused.

This exploration is for those who love yoga but aren't sure how to avoid appropriation and respect its roots. It's also for those who have caused harm and want to make things better. It is for those who recognize, feel the pain, resonate and are finding and building their voices and capacities.

You may respond to it differently depending on your positionality. Whether you are South Asian, Black, Indigenous, Person of Color or white. This is part of the relative truth of our experience. Where you may hear perspectives that are different than yours you can utilize it to help deepen your empathy.

Through our informative and exploratory reflections, you'll be guided to explore your connection to yoga while learning how to properly honor and not appropriate in your practice.

These explorations lead us to the true aim of yoga personally and socially—that of complete unity.

You may find this to be a deep inner journey of self-reflection and growth as well as an outer journey of change and taking on new practices.

You'll learn key skills to help you understand the complex world of cultural issues in yoga and deepen your connection to yoga practice.

Practicing yoga by embracing yoga's roots and exploring the breadth and depth of the practice, as well as its inspiration to serve others, is an invitation. It is an invitation to choose connection over separation. To trust and find deep ancestral wisdom we have inside us thundering through like a roaring train or rustling like sweet grass in the soft wind.

Yoga is a lifelong reminder that we cannot help but live and breathe beautiful connection to our innate personal and ancestral wisdom.

HONOR (DON'T APPROPRIATE) YOGA: WHY WE MUST EMBRACE YOGA'S ROOTS NOW

It was a normal day. I awoke with the sun, practiced gratitude and prayer and had just finished my yoga and meditation practice. I sat down at my desk and opened my laptop. A message came through the top of my inbox about a big international yoga event.

Excited, I checked out the headliners and teachers. I saw face after face. And was struck with a shocking realization. I felt queasy as I saw not one teacher of color, not one of size, not one trans teacher, not one who didn't fit the "norm" of what yoga has come to be in the West.

My stomach sank. The positive energy from my morning practice evaporated.

This wasn't a surprise. I'd been seeing yoga festivals, trainings, workshops, schools and institutions just like these for decades. This was the norm.

As someone from India and Britain, with the roots of yoga so deep in my own culture, I had many questions. And I didn't hesitate to ask them.

I wrote to these festivals, events, schools and asked them why, when yoga comes from India and has roots in thousands of years of practice and expertise cultivated by Brown and Black people, there are so few, or none, to be found in their event?

Almost no one answered but when they did reply the answers I received were not often receptive. Those who did answer said they only brought on speakers with large followings as this was how they did things and necessary for their bottom line.

I wrote to Kirtan and yoga-focused music festivals, excited for them to foreground the talented South Asian musicians I know. After weeks of waiting, I got the answer that the musicians didn't have a big enough following.

Then, another festival wrote back that the proposed South Asian artists' music was too authentic and wouldn't appeal to a wide audience.

I wrote to well-known yoga festivals to ask them to hire, "platform"—by which I mean, provide platforms for or otherwise promote teachers from marginalized groups—spotlight any and all of the Black, Indigenous, or South Asian teachers who have been teaching authentic yoga traditions and practices for about a decade. Silence or rejection were again the results.

These responses felt like silent barbs in an already-open wound. One after another, the rejections rolled in.

I began to see a pattern. One negative response may be a coincidence. Or a marketing issue. But year after year, when festivals, summits, conferences and events invite only some people in and, in effect, block those in marginalized groups, we have to ask the hard questions.

Why aren't some people, and some teachings, being listened to, uplifted and given platforms? Why is what we know as yoga in the West so watered down and so far from the roots a full practice offers?

It dawned on me: because this is not one person's fault. It is a system at play. This is normative culture in action.

The tricky thing is that almost no one realizes they are upholding a system that includes some and excludes others. It's not intentional. But it is happening. And there may be some people doing this consciously. But most people are not conscious of the exclusivity they are creating. By putting people who look like them on the expert lineup, they feel justified in their positionality as expert in a field that did not originate with them.

And it can be changed.

I wrote my usual questions to that big yoga event in an email and hit send.

I closed my computer and sat in the dappled sunlight coming through the window, shining on the altar next to my desk. Suddenly, after many years of waiting for replies, I got a bolt of inspiration.

Instead of asking, waiting and hoping for a future to be different, for more of us to be welcomed into the spotlight, why not create the platform ourselves?

I realized in that moment, I have the power. You have the power too. No matter how many moments we've not acted, or done harmful things or missed an opportunity, we can choose in each new moment to move in the direction of equity and inclusivity.

You truly have the power to create diverse spaces. You have the ability to learn the depth of what yoga has to offer us. To learn from, uplift and share the many faces of ancient and modern wisdom. To hear from the indigenous knowledge-keepers and way-showers of yoga today.

These actions support all of us. Yoga practitioners, teachers and seekers who are curious about or wish to be part of this movement in embracing authentic yoga while at the same time creating equity in our world. They support the preservation of yoga practice for the future.

Fortunately, there is a framework that emerges from within the yoga tradition, itself, to help us do this work.

THE EMBRACE YOGA'S ROOTS FRAMEWORK: YOGIC SCIENCE OF SOCIAL JUSTICE

Within the yoga tradition are the tools we need in order to understand how to embrace the practice. The practice of the limbs of yoga is the path of learning to embrace yoga's roots and not to diminish, water down or appropriate. This may be a process of unlearning some of what you have learned as well as relearning a different path and process.

Just as we aim to move beyond diversity to equity, we go beyond simply doing what's sufficient to truly embracing the roots of yoga, in every aspect of our practice. Embracing yoga's roots is an invitation to explore what it means to be a vessel for yoga today.

This work is born from the seed in you that knows there is an essence to yoga that is far deeper than what we typically see.

This seed blooms from a determined truth; Whatever causes separation, within ourselves or with others, is not yoga. Whatever leads us toward unity is yoga.

However, unity isn't some idealistic dream that we can just wish into being. Skipping over the often-divided reality we live within isn't the solution. Pretending separation and suffering doesn't exist is not the fastest way to unity.

This is why yoga naturally emerges as a science of social equality and justice. We must explore and understand all of the causes of separation, address them and realize the potential of yoga as unity.

This application of yoga to recognizing the dignity and worth of all beings was brought alive during the nonviolent revolution that freed India from British colonial rule. Application of yogic wisdom enabled the Indians to regain their ability to refuse colonial oppression, rule themselves, and at the same time not dehumanize the colonizers.

In *Patanjali's Yoga Sutra* verse 2.22, we understand the importance of practicing to serve our own and others' liberation.

2.22 KRTĀRTHAM PRATI NASTAM APY ANASTAM TAD ANYA SĀDHĀRANATVAT.

Freedom arises when we see things as they are and can remain at ease and calm with what is. Conscious of the causes of separation and illusion that exist the world over, we understand our shared human condition. We work for ourselves and for others to create liberation for ourselves and for all beings, our siblings, to create human uplift in this world.

The path of embracing yoga's roots inspired me to create the Honor (Don't Appropriate) Yoga Summit, an online interview series where I interviewed over 40 diverse experts in 2019. The Honor (Don't Appropriate) Yoga Summit has, to date, had two powerful seasons. The first season foregrounded majority BIPOC speakers on the importance of diversity in Western yoga spaces. The second season featured South Asian/Desi vital voices in yoga today. With this summit my vision was to change the Western yoga landscape, share wisdom from many incredible teachers of color who are often excluded, and expand the scope of conversations on yoga in the West. With over 10,000 participants and counting, we are continuing to shift the terrain and conversation of yoga today as well as learning from diverse perspectives and voices. In creating this project, I began to transform into who I was seeking. The work of embracing yoga's roots can transform you as well as you develop your relationship with yoga as unity.

The key to addressing the problem lies within the practice of yoga itself. To realize unity in ourselves and in yoga, we must recognize the need for more inclusive practices and spaces. We can no longer ignore the things that divide us or keep us apart. No matter how many times we say, "We are all one," or "Everything is light and love," separation, injustice and division will remain all around us.

Unity doesn't mean erasing or ignoring someone's reality or lived experience simply for the sake of "being one" or staying "positive." Here, we mean uniting our humanity while understanding the many systems that oppress.

The key is that these divisions often are centered on the things that make us unique or different. We must look at what separates us and bring it to light so we can address it. Yogic tools such as *svadhyaya* (self-inquiry), *ahimsa* (kindness) and *satya* (truthfulness) will help us understand and evolve this process.

What we think separates us can perhaps more authentically bring us together, not in a way that erases our differences, but one that embraces them.

This book is divided into four key steps in the process of creating equity and unity.

Each part is an important step in the growth-oriented process and framework that will help us go beyond just honoring yoga to embracing yoga's roots.

We will take these steps together.

First, we will address the blocks to unity and causes of **separation** by looking deeply at the source of our cultural suffering.

Next, we will understand separation through **reflection**, exploring all the ways it shows up on our mats, in our studios, and in our practices and lives.

Then, we will practice the path of unity as **reconnection through action**, taking steps toward repair, healing, reparations, unity, living and embracing yoga.

Finally, we will learn to embody our yoga as **liberation**, unity with self and others.

The aim with embracing yoga's roots is practicing yoga as a means of inclusive, nonhierarchical spirituality.

Yoga as a framework of social justice gives us the tools, the framework and the practices to root out separation, oppression and exclusion in the various social structures in which we may find ourselves.

It is important to address that yoga itself is separate from religion, though it has coexisted along with many. Yoga emerged within Śramaṇa, or renunciate, traditions, according to Yoga in Śramana Tradition by N. K. Jain. In an attempt to find liberation from suffering through spiritual endeavors, yoga practices emerged and were practiced and codified amongst different schools and styles of practitioners.

Yoga is separate from any religion even though it has been utilized by different religions. It is important to name and call out when yoga itself is used as a tool to oppress. This text seeks to address yoga in the West. It is also important to assert that this work is not intended to advocate or advance a Casteist or Hindutva attempt to claim that all yoga is Hindu and then use yoga as a tool of oppression and exclusion. This type of co-opting of yoga for separation and division also necessitates disruption and interruption as does caste based oppression.

Yoga is not under the purview of any one religion, but developed alongside Śramana traditions that emerged as Jain and Buddhist as well as Vedic and Hindu traditions and later was influenced by Islam and Christianity. Yoga does not belong exclusively to any one religion and an explanation of this is more than we will cover in the scope of this book.

Whether we are acting for Black Lives Matter, Anti-Caste discrimination, or equal rights for oppressed folks around the world, yoga supports us with tools, a framework and practices to undo separation and create equity and unity.

Yoga is here for us to uplift, learn and embrace a practice of empathy and spiritual democracy.

SEPARATION

So many things contribute to our suffering and separation. Cultural appropriation and disconnection can come only from a place of separation. Harm is caused all around. We will examine, using a yogic framework, the roots of big concepts such as racism and oppression so we can break them down, understand them and change them.

REFLECTION

In order to live yoga as unity, we must explore and understand the tools of separation and look closely at the practices and tools that got us to a place of separateness. When we look them squarely in the eye, even if that eye is our own, we can begin to dismantle them, as well as set the stage for yoga as liberation.

RECONNECTION THROUGH ACTION

Once we see clearly the causes of separation, we can change our habits and practices, our thoughts, words and actions to be more in line with our true intention of unity. With a focus on repair, healing and reparations, we can develop the tools to truly live and embrace yoga and achieve true unity.

LIBERATION

Liberation is what the yogic path has always been about. We find that when we return again to the path of yoga and practice a full expression of it, we have all the tools we need to live a liberatory life for ourselves and others. This is the union that is fully possible with a deep yoga practice.

This is a growth-oriented system that follows the teachings of yoga itself. There is no way to fail at this process other than to stop trying. Keep going, returning again, reflecting deeper and acting in different ways. You will inevitably find and create more true unity in your world.

QUESTIONS TO SUPPORT THE EMBRACE YOGA'S ROOTS FRAMEWORK

Based on the classical texts of yoga such as the *Bhagavad Gita* and *Patanjali Yogashastra*, as well as contemporary social justice organizing and work, I have developed a foundational framework that emerges from within the yoga tradition to support us in knowing if we are embracing yoga. Yoga is inherently a science of social justice that leads to liberation for ourselves and others, collectively. It is a systematically organized body of knowledge on human liberation.

To practice this science we can ask ourselves: What is the essence of yoga as *yuj*, as unity? With this framework as a guide, you can deepen your practice to get closer to that essence.

As we go through the book, the following questions underpin everything through which you will be guided. You can always ask yourself these questions to see if you are embracing yoga.

1. **Is it causing Separation?** Is it Unsafe? Harmful? Safe? Kind?
   Practice *ahimsa*, non-harm and kindness.

2. **Am I embracing roots?** Consider whether you are embracing yoga's roots and lineage, as well as your own roots.
   Practice *vichara* and *satya*, wisdom, deep listening and speaking your truth.

3. **Does this action create connection?** To yourself? To others? For a group?
   Practice *yoga* as *tapas* by taking action to uplift others.

4. **Does it lead to unity and liberation?** Does it make you and/or others more mindful, free, peaceful, powerful or calm? Does it contribute to systemic change for human uplift?
   Practice yoga as unity for *samadhi* to create liberation for all.

This work is the yogic science of social justice and application of yogic philosophy in our times. It is about relationship, and it invites a willingness to connect. We embody a spirit of learning and trying and embrace conversations and discussions across differences.

By listening and applying the Embrace Yoga's Roots framework to your own actions and practice, you will go far toward embracing yoga and creating a life of more peace, calm, freedom and joy for yourself and others.

A NOTE ON CULTURAL APPROPRIATION AND WHITE SUPREMACY

In this book, you will see me use *Sanskrit.* I will also talk about cultural appropriation. I describe what cultural appropriation is and provide examples, ways to avoid it, ways to repair harm caused and what to do instead.

Sanskrit is a specific and precise language with powerful resonance. Each sound has embedded within it the essence of the meaning of yoga itself. It is important to use the original language used at the time when yoga was first organized into a system or way of being in relationship with one's self and the world.

I will talk about race, white supremacy, representation, reparations and other topics which I will define and discuss throughout the book. There is also a glossary at the end for easy reference.

If some of these terms—such as colonization, patriarchy or white supremacy—are new to you, or you don't fully understand what they mean, don't worry. I will explain them and provide examples to help you recognize these ideas and behaviors.

Knowledge is power. And with this power we can create change.

There is, in my understanding, no way to separate the issues of cultural appropriation and systems of oppression.

Cultural appropriation is a byproduct of colonization and empire.

Colonization and empire depend on hierarchical systems of oppression, such as patriarchy and white supremacy, to function.

These systems work across all our social institutions, from political to social to cultural to spiritual.

To repair the harm done to yoga—the harms of oppression and cultural appropriation—we need to address the root causes of separation and disconnection. And we need to address the systems that create and perpetuate harm.

We will examine and discuss all of it, holding close to our heart the possibility for yoga in its fullness—for oneness, unity and complete liberation from suffering for all beings.

Perhaps this is an ambitious aim. Sometimes healing the harm of oppressive systems feels far away or hard to imagine.

But our deep listening and our imaginations can liberate us.

By undertaking this exploration, we not only honor yoga we embrace it, we can also co-create new systems that function on connection, with love, care and intersectionality, and contribute to a unity that is possible for us all.

WHAT THE EMBRACE YOGA FRAMEWORK IS NOT

The practice of embracing the roots of yoga is a science and, inherently, an engaged equity practice.

This is not a complete Yoga Teacher Training (YTT), though I strongly believe this material should be required curriculum in every YTT program.

This is not a yoga philosophy course. You will find some philosophy in practice but will not find in-depth teachings on *yama* or *niyama* (yogic ethics), *asana* (poses), *pranayama* (breathwork), *dharana* (focus), *dhyana* (meditation) and *samadhi* (liberation), *tapas*, (yogic discipline), *mantra* (sacred sound), *mudra* (sacred gesture) or a comprehensive exploration of yoga philosophy or history. These topics are best transmitted orally, as my teacher has done for me, and teachers have done throughout the ages. These topics are explored in my online courses as well as during in-person workshops. Toward the end of the book, we will explore some concrete ways to deepen your yoga *sadhana* (practice).

This exploration is created for you to do the work. It is specifically designed for self-reflective exploration and a growth process of embracing unity and equity in yoga.

I will be guiding you to explore the work of embracing and not appropriating yoga. To examine the social norms and constructs that you've helped erect in yoga in the West. To learn, name and dismantle the systems that keep us stuck in separation. If you find yourself triggered then take care of yourself and continue to re-engage.

This work is not conclusive, nor does it comprehensively address every problematic issue in our yoga spaces.

Reading this is not an exemption to examine one's own social conditioning. Nor is it a permission slip to say that you are done doing the work. This work is continuous and ever-evolving. Exploring one's biases and gaps and seeking out yoga teachers from within the tradition as well as anti-racism educators must be part of the equity work for anyone serious about embracing yoga's roots.

For those of you reading closely, yes, in many ways the yoga philosophy mentioned above and the framework of Embracing Yoga are one and the same, as I hope you will find during our journey through this work and in your life as you apply these tools and practices.

II
TOOLS AND BEST PRACTICES

"Each human being is both unique and universal. When the two things get integrated, it is that you call a fulfilled human being, one who has been able to realize the discords, overcome them, and make of him or herself as single home...

There is no conflict at all between the great developments of science and technology and the true religious sense of wisdom or spirituality. It is essential to coordinate and integrate these great instruments for the purpose of human welfare."

—Dr. S. Radhakrishnan, *Faith Renewed*

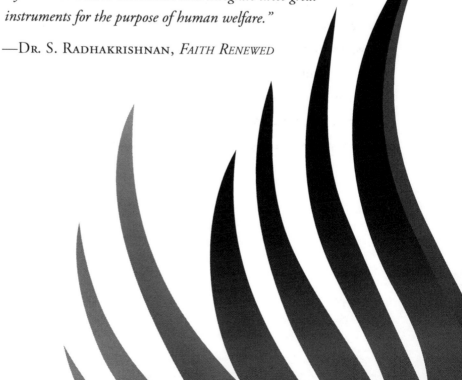

TOOLS FOR THE PATH OF PRACTICE: WHAT YOU WILL NEED

YOGA IN ACTION INCLUDES EVOLVING PRACTICES FOR SELF-REFLECTION, self-care and community care. We can employ some best practices in this work toward unity.

PRACTICES FOR REFLECTION

We are embarking together on a process of seeing what is often unseen. What a beautiful journey inquiry can be! Reflection can allow new insights to arise. Reflection is often the gateway to embodiment. With time, care and attention toward deep reflection, the roots of yoga will inhabit every corner of your life.

As we do this work and explore together, a lot will come up. It will be helpful to have a way or place to process. This is *svadhyaya*, or self-inquiry, in action.

Grab a pen and paper or recorder, and find a place to think, speak, emote or write. I have included prompts for reflection throughout the book. I've intentionally titled them "reflection questions" rather than "writing prompts" to be inclusive of those who learn differently and who may want to record, think, speak, discuss with others or in some other way engage with and process this work.

If you are writing, here are some suggestions:
- Keep a journal of a size, shape or texture you like.
- Use a pen or pencil you are drawn to.
- Create ritual around your writing.
- Write at a similar time each day, for example, first thing in the morning before *asana* and meditation, at lunch or before bed.
- Allow yourself to write without censoring yourself and let your thoughts flow freely.

If you are reflecting by thinking, recording or speaking, here are some suggestions:

- Find a sacred space to do this reflection.
- Reflect at a similar time each day.
- Create a ritual around reflection.
- Allow yourself to create a safe and sacred space for your reflection to flow freely.

In general, whether you write, speak, think, record or something else, you'll be aided by a perspective of progress and not perfection. It's not about doing the work perfectly. Or about understanding every little thing. It is enough to be here. To start, to stop, reflect and, always, to continue.

PRACTICES FOR SELF-CARE

To do this work together we need many resources. Among the resources that can support us are practices for self-care and community care.

As we undertake this exploration together, I invite you to continue to nourish yourself, within, beyond and all around the work. Melissa A. Fabello (2015) of Everyday Feminism defines self-care as, "any set of practices that makes you feel nourished, whether that's physically, emotionally, spiritually, all of the above."

As we move forward, the following qualities may be helpful:

- **A reflective mind and heart.** Notice emotions and feelings, and when you experience resistance, be willing to explore a bit deeper. When we move through resistance we often uncover impactful insights.

- **Curiosity.** It helps to get curious. Ask questions. Get curious within your own experience, as well as with the world around you.

- **Holding Tension.** When doing important work, triggers and tension can arise. It can help to develop practices to remain present while you hold the tension. Yoga *asana* is an incredible practice that guides us in growing our skills of holding tension. Imagine holding a rubber band between both hands. The right amount of tension feels engaged. Too much, and the band breaks. Too little and it sags. This can give purpose to our yoga *asana* practice.

  It is an art to hold tension. It often can feel like we are being squeezed in many directions when we do this type of work. So many different thoughts and feelings come up. Family members, studios, friends and loved ones may feel differently than you or may not understand. Having supportive and inquisitive people around you on parallel journeys can be helpful.

  Teo Drake, spiritual activist, queer-identified yoga teacher and artisan has shared some words to support us with this practice. "When you shift into discomfort, it allows me to shift out of pain."

  Holding tension allows you to sit in the entirety of your experience—pleasant, unpleasant, neutral—and allow the wisdom of simply being there to let new actions and awareness unfold.

- **Grief.** Holding space for grief is a part of the process of working for justice and liberation. There can be so much sadness in acknowledging how far we are from the world in which you may wish us to be. As I have learned from my siblings in past liberation struggles, such as the anti-apartheid movement in South Africa, the Independence Movement in India, the Peace Movement in Vietnam and the U.S., there can be so much grief at facing and working with the struggles for equality all around us. Being present to this grief, holding it, as we would a child in our care, can bring tenderness and care.

- **Anger.** Making time and space for anger and sacred rage is part of the process. There is space for righteous and sacred rage against all that has been taken, erased and lost. And from this rage can be born the truth, healing, and reclaiming that needs to occur.

- **Trust.** No one has authority over your truth and your ancestry but you. This is something that's taken me a while to understand. We all have epistemic authority over our own experience.

- **Self-Appreciation.** Acknowledge and celebrate yourself.

- **Growth Mindset.** Appreciate that you are learning.

- **Rest.** Space for sleep—naps, *yoga nidra*, body scanning, *shavasana*, and meditation may all be helpful. However you rest, invite it in.

- **Flexibility.** As you do this work, give yourself space to be flexible, to take the time to inquire as to what you need. Be patient with how you engage with this work. You may need to step away from this book for a time and take care of yourself.

- **Embodiment.** Process, move, sing, write, connect and discuss. Then come back to the work. Allow time for integration and reflection. Don't expect the process to always look the same or to be linear. Get into your body. Move, drum, sing, dance, lay on the grass. Know that what it looks like for you from one moment to the next might change. What it looks like for a colleague or friend may be different than for you. Open and create space for the entire process as it evolves and deepens.

- **Commitment.** Return to this practice. Underneath the challenges and growth lies the truth of all of our connection. When you return to this work, you are returning to that truth of deep interconnectedness and belonging that yoga offers us.

PRACTICES FOR COMMUNITY CARE

We can do this work alone and we can also find immense support when we do it in community. Connecting with others can support us as well as amplify our impact. Neither method is superior or inferior. Both are welcome. I'm offering suggestions for community care here in the spirit of how our liberation is inextricably linked.

Community care is about how we contribute to others.

Often our healing isn't linear—we don't have to heal ourselves first before we help others. In fact, through working and growing in community we, ourselves, experience moments of liberation.

Many queer folks of color are paving the way in this work of community care. It is no accident, because communities most impacted by oppression have needed to form systems for self- and community sustenance. Cara Page, Alejandra Tobar Alatriz, Anjali Taneja, Telesh Lopez, Susan Raffo and Yashna Padamsee have all been at the forefront of this work for National Healing Justice. "It is our responsibility not as individuals, but as communities to create structures in which self-care changes to community care. In which we are cared-for and able to care for others" (Padamsee, 2011).

When we care for one another we enable networks of transformation to multiply within us and all around us. Neuroplasticity is the idea that we can change our habits because of the ability to essentially rewire our brains through creating change. Neurons that fire together, wire together—according to an idea originated by psychologist Donald Hebb in 1949. It has been further developed by many psychologists who point to the potential of the human mind to define, redefine and shape itself (Ackerman, 2018).

We can expand this notion of growth and change beyond one brain to many. I like to think of this as if we are in the process of creating "culturalasticity" (Barkataki, 2015).

Communities that heal, grow, care and inspire together, wire together, and bring us all higher together.

You can host informal discussion group circles, practicing the yogic practices of deep listening and loving speech and explore the reflection questions and concepts in this book together.

Note: If you do engage this work in community, please practice *asteya* (non-stealing) and uplift one another in a culture of connection. Cite sources and ensure that each participant purchases their own copy of this book.

ENGAGING THE COMMUNITY

You are more than welcome to engage this work in ways that are most supportive for you.

If you like, you can seek out friends, studio spaces, communities, support groups, communities with shared values, along with those interested in exploring what you care to explore.

Here are some practices to support community care:

- **Reach out.** Connect to others, form discussion groups or learning circles. Check in with one another. Call, message or text.

- **Co-regulate support.** Ask and receive support, such as getting consent to place your hand on someone's back if they need support grounding themselves, or having someone watch your kids or pick up food from the store for you to allow you more time and space for this work.

- **Create *ahimsa*-focused space.** Create space for sustained acts of kindness and compassion. For example, creating cultures where folks take care of their own bodies, where support for caring for one another is normal and celebrated, goes a long way to creating a culture of care. *Ahimsa*-focused space can be created when the community is dedicated to "safe and brave space guidelines" as offered here, when transparency and authenticity are cultivated and care and inclusion for different perspectives are honored.

- **Gather.** Allow the way and form of community care to shift and evolve, such as neighborhood groups, communal homes, support groups, service or activist groups and friend circles.

Additionally, I have an Embrace Yoga Collective online group you can join if you'd like a collaborative place to discuss this work.

Ultimately, your interweaving web of self-reflection, self-care and community care creates a powerful foundation for exploring and living yoga ethics.

DEEP ENGAGEMENT

Whether you work individually, in community or in some combination, the Embrace Yoga framework is intentionally created to take you through a specific process to bring us toward embodiment of yoga as unity. First, we will address the causes of separation and reflect on the ways they may show up in our lives and practice. Then we will reconnect through action and move toward a liberatory practice of yoga as unity.

This process is presented with an intentional structure. Ideally, you will read and work through the book from start to finish.

A REMINDER OF 3 KEYS FOR SUCCESS

1. **Reflect**

   Take time to really reflect on these ideas and bring them alive. Revisit the tools for reflection as discussed above as many times as you need.

2. **Intent: Be Open to Learning and Seeing Things in a New Way**

   The first section focuses on education, defining terms and concepts and encouraging self-reflection. This section is linear and logical. There are concepts to understand, questions on which to reflect and actions to take. Your work in this section builds a foundation for the material and work that follow as we move into more practice-oriented application of yoga as unity.

3. **Respect the Process. Notice Triggers. Take Breaks if Needed and Keep Going**

   Pauses are welcome. But no matter what, keep going. It is critical for the future of yoga that you are here.

BEST PRACTICES FOR COURAGEOUS CONVERSATIONS: BRAVE AND SACRED SPACE

('From Safe Spaces to Brave Places: A New Way to Frame Dialogue Around Diversity and Social Justice,' 2013 by Brian Arao and Kristi Clemens)

This work of yoga is divine and it is sacred. I will share here the guidelines for discussion that I use when I facilitate. I use these guidelines to create powerful and intimate containers for transformation in workshops or speaking events. Even with hundreds of people, you'd be surprised at the intimacy a shared container built on trust can provide. With a container like this, the space is set to do the deep, reflective and even uncomfortable work necessary for embracing yoga.

In our context in this book, I'm inviting you to hold these guidelines and perhaps invite in other guidelines for yourself.

DEEP READING AND INTENTION SETTING

We can read in so many ways—to consume, attack, argue, deflect, learn, connect. Can you set an intention to stay open-minded and positively present? Each time you open the book, as you read, I invite you to try creating a small ritual for yourself that invokes deep reading.

Perhaps take three deep breaths. Light a candle. Tune in through your special way and take in these words from a heart-centered place.

REFLECTION QUESTIONS

Throughout the book you will find descriptive sections followed by questions for reflection. When you write, speak, reflect, discuss or journal in response to your reflection questions, please find your way of tuning into your heart. Take a moment, perhaps even placing one hand on your heart, and listen for that deeper voice of inner truth.

And then begin. And begin again.

BRAVE SPACE GUIDELINES

The guidelines shared below were inspired by the concept for Brave Space Guidelines as developed by Brian Arao and Kristi Clemens in 'From Safe Spaces to Brave Places: A New Way to Frame Dialogue Around Diversity and Social Justice,' 2013.

GUIDELINES

- Speak from the heart
- Listen deeply from the heart
- Respect
- Take risks, lean in to growth, feel and grant permission to be messy
- Keep respectful confidentiality when you are in conversation with others

MIND-BODY LEARNING / CHECK IN WITH BODY AND BREATH

- Self-reflect. Process with patience, self-care, self-love and respect
- Use "I" statements when speaking with others, especially about charged or otherwise challenging topics and emotions
- Make space / Take space
- Strive to embody a Growth Mindset—Know "I am not my own or others' mistakes"; "I'm willing to learn, grow and change. I see that others can, also."

HOLD AWARENESS OF MULTIPLE TRUTHS

- Simultaneity (both/and): Your and my truth can contradict and coexist
- Be willing to hear someone else's truth as different from yours
- Hold awareness of Intent vs. Impact
- Reflect rather than fix others

CONTEXT

- Bring your whole self, even the unhealed or unexamined parts of yourself
- Reflect and notice your own positionality, privilege, power and allyship
- Hold awareness and willingness to own or speak up around microaggressions when appropriate

EMBRACE THE HEALING PROCESS. OPEN TO LISTENING. CONFLICT IS NATURAL AND OKAY.

- Triggers are normal and natural in this process

- Own, name, speak when it is right for you (often your words are what someone else needs to hear, too)
- Ask for support—from self, one-on-one, from group, wider communities and mentors

With these guidelines we seek to offer best practices for creating and holding brave spaces that minimize harm, knowing that not all spaces are safe for all. We do our best to uplift all beings. These guidelines are a work in progress and a living document and are always open to improvement. These guidelines are created alongside and influenced by Thich Nhat Hanh and the Plum Village Community, Cleveland Humanities Magnet teaching team and the community of Diasporas in LA.

REFRAMING SANKALPA: EQUITY IS IMPACT OVER INTENTION

There is no perfect translation for the Sanskrit word *sankalpa* into English. It is something like caring for intention and impact.

In modern yoga in the West we are often great at setting intentions. We set intentions at the beginning of practice. When we forget, we slip it in at the end of *asana* practice. Sometimes we make an intention at both the beginning and the end of practice.

Let's explore: What is your *sankalpa*—your deep, heartfelt, soul-level intention for doing this work?

Sankalpa goes beyond just intention. *Sankalpa* truly cares for impact. This framework helps us create equity in yoga by considering what impact you are having. What impact do you have when you are taking or running a yoga class, studio, retreat or training?

Remember that intention does not equal impact. So yes, set your intention, but don't stop there. Care for your impact. Impact is how you show up; how your presence, your action, your intention lands.

How does it impact and interact with others, including those who may not be in the room? As you consider, know that the world needs you to help yoga become more inclusive and diverse.

As you create your Embrace Yoga *sankalpa,* consider your intention and also care for your impact.

REFLECTION QUESTIONS

- What is your *sankalpa* for doing this work?

- What is the impact or possible impacts it may create?

- What are the moral and social implications on the people, communities and ecosystems you impact, as well as practical and useful implications of your personal intention?

"Someone, somewhere, needs to take courage to break the cycle of violence. Forgiveness is superior to justice. Being kind and compassionate to those who are good to you is easy. True forgiveness and compassion come only when one is able to forgive even those who have committed barbaric acts. If the terrorist Angulimala is capable of renouncing violence, then tell me, is your civilized society also capable of being truly civilized and renouncing violence?"

—Satish Kumar, *The Buddha and the Terrorist*

III
SEPARATION

"Do every action you must do
And do not be attached to your actions' fruits.
Self-possessed, resolute, act without any thought of results,
open to success or failure.
This equanimity is yoga.
Do not be attached to inaction.
This skill in action is yoga."

—Bhagavad Gita 2.47

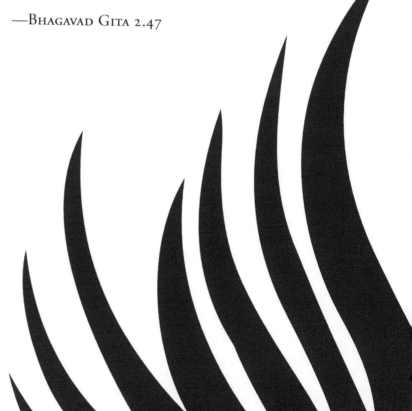

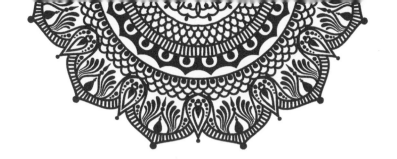

PART 1

CONTEXT

"Even if you have known the real truth,
you have to practice always."

— Yoga Vasistha, 10.21

A BRIEF YOGA HISTORY

Yoga is an organized group or science of physical, mental and spiritual disciplines that originated in ancient India in an oral tradition that potentially predates the *Vedas*, India's oldest-known spiritual scriptures.

Yoga is a practice that comes from the subcontinent of India and has been practiced, passed down, codified and developed for somewhere between 2,500 and 10,000 years. We don't know the exact dates for when yoga was first practiced. Based on more recent research, Western scholars are dating yoga to around the time of the Buddha, some 2,500 years ago (Powell, 2018).

However, many *sanyasis* and villagers I interviewed during a research trip to India claimed that yoga has been practiced, developed and shared for thousands of years before that (Barkataki, 2009).

This question around dating the practice calls up our "epistemology," or how we know what we know.

Throughout history, various groups in India—across religions (Hindu, Jain and Buddhist) and other cultures—have defined yoga according to differing beliefs and goals.

What is undisputed is that yogic practices sprung up in an Indic culture that respected and learned from nature and deeply valued spiritual exploration. Where practitioners were found in forests, caves, beside rivers, on the outskirts of villages and cities, devoting their life to the exploration of how to relieve suffering and find liberation through daily moments in deep practice.

It is with great honor and respect that we have this practice that has been developed and passed down from teacher to student to be here with us today.

Now, yoga is expanding to become a global phenomenon. In this light, yoga describes both an optimal unitive state of consciousness, and the techniques, philosophies, practices and lifestyles that bring one to a unified state. Various yoga lineages, styles, schools and traditions vary in approach, vision and goals. Yoga may be utilized for many different means. We need to be mindful of where yoga may be used for fundamentalist, nationalistic, cult or abusive means.

Many define it differently. Some teachers situate it within a religious context and specify that yoga creates a merging with the divine so deeply that you become divine. Others are decidedly secular and say that yoga is a practice that helps us uncover the divinity within us. These differences and tensions are not new to yoga and modern-day discussions over the varying definitions and practices of yoga mirror its syncretic roots.

Most definitions of yoga have in common a teaching on union. Just as we are all the same as the Universal, you and I are also not separate or different in our innermost being.

We ourselves may have had this experience in the depth of meditation, or after a powerful yoga *asana* class, where you feel completely at home, one with all, immersed in the unity of just being.

This is the experience of yoga, however fleeting.

This understanding of yoga as unity can also invite us to bring this alive in our day-to-day lives. From meditation or practice on our mat to welcoming people into our studios and classrooms, we can practice yoga as unity.

We can also remind ourselves of the Embrace Yoga framework and ask ourselves, is my behavior causing separation rather than unity? Is that separation rooted in willful ignorance, cognitive dissonance, or bypassing a harsh reality I'm not willing to confront? Can I remember the divinity in all as my own *and* understand each one of us has a different lived experience?

These questions can be our yoga unity check-in as we bring this practice of yoga as unity into our personal, family, community and social world.

REFLECTION QUESTIONS

- What do you know about yoga history and how do you know it?

- Are you using a colonizer's measuring stick or an ancestor's measuring stick to measure and assess truth claims about yoga's history?

- What specifically in yoga history do you want to learn more about?

YOGA'S MODERN HISTORY: FROM SEPARATION TO LIBERATION

Yoga has always been a science of liberation. It is a coherent method for personal freedom, social justice and equity that has been tested over time and in practice.

Though it has often been reduced to little more than just carrying around a yoga mat and rolling it out to do a class where you move your body into different shapes, it is so much more.

Yoga is a complex and comprehensive system of specific practices of body, mind and spirit that guide the individual and society toward liberation and freedom from suffering.

Yoga is a mind, body and spiritual practice that invites deeper breath and presence through movement aligned with breath. It is a powerful practice and its potential for liberation is immense.

Much of the Indian Independence Movement was inspired and fueled by yoga applied to principles of nonviolent struggle and self-rule. Gandhi, one of the leaders of the Independence Movement, took the *Bhagavad Gita* to jail with him and used the *Gita's* yogic philosophy to fuel the methods used to create the foundations for independence. Throughout this trying time in India's history, yoga and yogis were instrumental in creating a culture of independence and justice.

When, under colonization in the late 18th century, the yogis in Northern India used their role and powers to address colonial domination, the British didn't take this dissidence lightly. The yogis were spiritual, as well as strategic. The yogis practiced not just spiritual disobedience, by daring to state that they were capable of ruling themselves, but civil disobedience. They would essentially practice by day, then at night come together and throw a wrench in the mechanisms of empire.

When I lived in Bihar, India, I heard many stories of how the yogis would actually disrupt the trains and trade routes of the British East India Company, so the goods they were exploiting could not get to their intended destination. This was an intentionally symbolic, as well as practical, disruption on the part of the yogis. They were, effectively, hitting the company where it hurt—in their pocketbook. They sought to make it "not worth it" to stay and colonize India. Though it would be two more centuries before British rule ended, the roots of Indian Independence are seeded in these yogis' actions.

"So powerful were these armed ascetics that throughout the final decades of the eighteenth century the British found themselves pitted against a yogi insurgency that would come to be known as the Sanyasi and Fakir Rebellion," researcher David Gordon White (2012) writes in *Yoga the Art of Transformation.*

Yogis formed groups focused on disrupting unfair control by empire. In the 1760s and 1770s, as reported in the Madras Courier (2017), spiritual practitioners known as Sanyasis and Fakirs (Hindu and Sufi renunciates, along with those of other undetermined faiths) banded together to undermine the rent control, feudal control and political control of the British East India Company.

The militant yogis won many battles against the empire, and disrupted trade routes. They were so successful that the British Raj outlawed yogis from entering certain parts of India (their own homelands). Though land and nature were key parts of yogic practice, the British response was to outlaw yogis from parts of the empire; that included the yogis' homes and sacred places. There were laws on the books in certain parts of India that made it illegal for a yogi or *sanyasi* to walk the streets in parts of Bihar, according to the villagers who live there. The British tactic of dehumanization was honed by over a century of domination over Black and Brown bodies. Recorded early 18th century descriptions of yogis were often as "degenerates engaging in sexual excesses or as weapon carrying mercenaries," White adds.

Often, the Colonial British responded with orientalist fascination or violent suppression to Indian yogic cultures.

Yogis, of course, persisted in their practices.

These strategies evolved over time into those employed by Gandhi and other nonviolent protestors who utilized yogic teachings such as *swadhyaya* (self-study) and *swadesh* (self-rule) to create self-control and autonomy to the extent that the British could no longer control the population they were forcefully oppressing. In effect, these early yogis helped contribute to the nonviolent yogic revolution that led to the Indian Independence.

The negative impacts of this colonization are far-reaching, as in many neo-colonial cultures, continuing today with the portrayals of young girls as brides, sex toys and generally objects for ownership by men. The colonized body goes on to colonize those it perceives as weaker than itself. This is perhaps one of the severest contemporary effects of colonization.

This leads us to locate ourselves in this inquiry. To ask about the legacy of yoga's roots, which themselves lie far before colonialism. **Is our practice liberating? Is it freeing? Does it disrupt oppression? Is it leading to greater freedom for ourselves and for others?**

We liberate by indigenizing meaning, returning the sovereignty of a practice to its roots, and from this foundation making meaning for ourselves. **We continue to indigenize meaning by returning the source of the knowledge to those from whom it has come.**

How does one create and sustain a liberatory yoga practice today?

One embraces yoga through a thoughtful, critical and intentionally decolonial practice that aligns with its core principles. (I will discuss colonialism and decolonization in detail in subsequent sections.)

We begin to embrace our practice when we humbly and respectfully consider yoga's history, context, its many branches and practices.

We can explore foundational yogic texts, such as *Patanjali's Yoga Sutras* as well as the *Bhagavad Gita,* in order to understand some of the principles underpinning these movements for liberation in the past as well as currently.

By doing this, we give ourselves a fighting chance at achieving yoga's aim: as *Yoga Sutra* 1.2 says, *"yogas chitta vritti nirodhah"*—freedom from the fluctuations of the mind, and enlightenment of mind, body and spirit.

Embracing yoga is the art of asking questions both on and off of our mats—of *living* a yoga of inquiry into truth and protest and change where there is separation.

Yoga practice is the science of personal liberation and social justice.

As with the yogis of the past, yoga can bring us liberation from every construct, including those of race, gender, time, space, location, identity and even history itself.

The practice of this liberating journey is one of creation. It is not a nationalistic promise of empire, or a regression, of "getting back" to a pure form of yoga which probably doesn't and never has existed, but rather a reclaiming, decolonizing and re-envisioning of its history and the current moment.

REFLECTION QUESTIONS

- Is our practice liberatory? Is it freeing?

- Does our yoga practice disrupt oppression?

- Does our practice lead to greater freedom for ourselves and for others?

S
E
P
A
R
A
T
I
O
N

HOW DO WE KNOW WHAT
WE KNOW ABOUT YOGA?

Many of my root teachers ask the same question in different ways. This is a question pointing to *vichara* or self-knowledge. One of my greatest teachers, Shankara, in Bihar, India, asks again and again, "How do you know what you know?"

Thich Nhat Hanh, Vietnamese Zen Buddhist monk and dear teacher, always asks me, "Are you sure?"

These questions point to a need for self-inquiry, practice, self-discovery and validation.

It is a compelling journey. We each search to understand for ourselves. And we can ask: What is authentic, liberating yoga? How do we understand what authentic yoga is when so much of it has come to us through a colonial lens? Can we actually locate it in ourselves in a culture so heavily built, informed and impacted by neo-colonialism and its equally oppressive twins, colonialism and capitalism?

Because these systems of complex power and oppression exist all around us and inform the very structures of our existence, what we can and must do is question, challenge and create new power structures.

It is a quest that invites the means to match the ends—that invites integrity in method and process. It invites us to ask the questions:

"Where do we find truth?"

And, "What is the truth yoga is asking of me?"

Is truth in our brains, in libraries, in historical texts, old documents, stories told by villagers and grandparents, on our yoga mats, in scholarly texts or in our hearts? It is, of course, in all these places. We might begin to ask, as we search for truth, which sources do we privilege over others?

It is a journey that invites us to our practice. To breathe, study, inquire within and without, to stay heart-centered and humble. A liberatory practice looks radically different for each person, especially if that person holds a marginalized identity.

Even in the ancient world, yoga practice was varied and non-standardized. Yoga *asana* was originally intended to prepare the body as a foundation for unity with the spirit (Mallinson, 2017).

Today, perhaps authentic practice is one that, such as in the time of the early *Vedas*, leads to deeper breath and space and freedom. Part of what an embracing yoga journey might feel like is being willing to understand, know, and feel the legacy and pain of colonization, usurpation, orientalization (the exotification of those from Eastern cultures), a complete obliteration of cultures and legacies and their subsequent replacements: globalization, media and consumer culture. As seekers, we can be accountable to honestly inquire about the impacts of this legacy of colonization on yoga and, therefore, on ourselves.

It is not about finding enemies or staying stuck in the past, but instead about honestly facing the impact of the past on the present and allowing ourselves, as well as the perpetrators of that violence, to be transformed.

It is about owning the ways that we, too, may be a part of all this. Asking, how are we complicit? It's about getting to interconnectedness and loving ourselves and our "enemies" enough to honestly transform one another. It is eruption into freedom, liberation, and the ability to question our own motives and those of our teachers. If we are sharing the practice of yoga for profit, how are we beholden to the marketplace, to our patrons/clients?

Are our intentions self-serving rather than reflective and giving?

Just like the motives the British were protecting when they tried to suppress the anti-colonial *sanyasis* and yogis to protect their financial interests and trade routes, today we find the yoga practice is co-opted, de-cultured, packaged, branded and currently in service of global capitalism. Are we able to separate the economic interests from the true inquiry and practice?

Let's ask the questions and do the research together. An eruption of equitable, liberating yoga is on the horizon. We explore separation, reflect, act for connection and finally, move toward and embrace liberation.

With a creative mindset, we can grow and build together, share a meaningful practice and take a stand for a new paradigm for the future of yoga.

REFLECTION QUESTIONS

What or who do you take as authority in your life?

Are there texts, books, teachers where you have found yogic wisdom?

Where in your own inner wisdom and body do you feel the resonance of the truth of yoga?

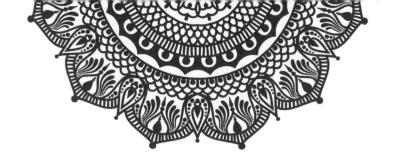

PART 2

YOGA AND CULTURAL APPROPRIATION

"Yoga became — and remains — a practice which allows western practitioners to experience the idea of another culture while focusing on the self."

— Shreena Gandhi and Lillie Wolff

As a culture, when we look at the causes of separation in yoga today, we need to begin with addressing cultural appropriation. When we explore and assess cultural appropriation, we are practicing *satya*, or truthfulness. When we interrupt appropriation, we are practicing *asteya*, or non-stealing.

Let's consider what is cultural appropriation and ask how it differs from cultural appreciation or honoring another culture.

The Oxford English Dictionary describes cultural appropriation as "the unacknowledged or inappropriate adoption of the customs, practices, ideas, etc. of one people or society by members of another and typically more dominant people or society."

There are two criteria that must be satisfied for there to be cultural appropriation when borrowing or using another's culture:

1. **Cultural appropriation involves power and dominance.**
2. **It involves doing emotional and psychological harm.**

Cultural appropriation is when someone uses someone else's culture, including practices, symbols, rituals, fashion or other elements from a target or "minority" culture, without considering the source, origins or people of that culture.

They may use another culture for various reasons, such as:

- To make a profit;
- To "make a new trend";
- To look cool or be fashionable;
- To be a cultural tourist or explore the "exotic";
- To mold another's culture into a more Eurocentric one (make it more Western or American so it is more palatable);
- A false perception of appreciation or alliance;
- Or for some other self-serving purpose without respecting or caring for the original culture, context or its people.

POWER, PRIVILEGE AND DOMINANCE

Cultural appropriation involves a dominant group with privilege and power taking from a marginalized group that has less systemic power. In modern history, colonizing powers, such as the British, used to take over the land of colonies then utilize and exploit the labor, natural resources, industrial power and anything deemed of value in that place.

Now, we don't have so much colonization of land or only physical resources, but instead, colonization of cultural informational wealth, such as we see with yoga. So those in the West still have more power, wealth, access, etc.

Groups in positions of power colonize a set of ideas and practices—in other words, cultural riches. This sector deals in information. It produces, manipulates, distributes and markets information products. It is taken and claimed by the dominant culture without credit to where it originated.

For example, a large US- or UK-based company that manufactures yoga leggings with images of deities printed on them is benefiting from the power imbalance that exists between India and the West through its economic and supremacist dominance.

Usually, this systemic imbalance of power involves exploitation. It includes the power to pick and choose what we take from a culture and leave the rest behind without regard for the impact on the communities affected or respect to its creators.

DOING HARM

Harm can come in two forms. One form of disrespect, for example, is taking a sacred deity or symbol and using it in a way that offends the person from the source culture.

Harm can also be material harm and is often inextricably linked to capitalism. Harm is material when the wellbeing of a person or group is negatively impacted by the appropriating actions. For example, this can happen when someone exploits the goods or labor of an Indian person and benefits from the labor without giving fair pay to the person who created the goods.

Often, when we take or borrow something from another culture, we think we are being innovative and adding flair or modern spice to our style. We are also under the belief that this is a way of acknowledging or expressing our appreciation of that culture. Without any understanding of the power dynamics at play, we don't realize there may be harm caused to folks who are in non-dominant positions or cultures.

It is important to understand that to truly combat cultural appropriation takes critical thinking. You'll need to consider some questions and ask *yourself* about appropriation, rather than look to an outside authority to determine answers for you. No one of us can speak for all of us. There is no final rule book.

In this book, I provide suggestions for methods of internal inquiry, including the reflection questions. What I hope we cultivate in this exploration is critical thinking.

CULTURAL APPROPRIATION IN YOGA

Cultural appropriation happens when a **dominant** group in a position of privilege and power politically, economically or socially adopts, benefits from, shares and even exploits the customs, practices, ideas or social and spiritual knowledge of another, usually **target** or **subordinate**, society or people (Barkataki, 2015).

Yoga is appropriated when a practice that has been developed over thousands of years to help humans overcome attachment and suffering is used to, for example, commodify, sell products and/or objectify the body. This happens frequently in modern culture, especially in the West.

For example:

When white-owned yoga studios display and sell Hindu or Indian cultural and religious iconography such as the *Om* symbol, *Ganesh* or *Lakshmi* statues, shirts, leggings, journals and so on, they are contributing to cultural appropriation.

Yoga students may not realize that wearing a cute *bindi* that matches their outfit or yoga leggings with *Om* or deities printed on them is also cultural appropriation.

Cultural appropriation causes harm when cultural norms, such as not placing symbols of the divine near the floor or by shoes, is blatantly disregarded—for instance, a statue of *Durga* or *Hanuman* sitting on the shoe rack at the entrance to class.

You can also read more about examples of cultural appropriation and how to practice cultural appreciation on my blog (www.susannabarkataki.

com/post/what-is-the-difference-between-cultural-appropriation-and-cul-tural-appreciation).

There are many places where cultural appropriation occurs in yoga. Two key concepts to help identify cultural appropriation are glamorization and sterilization, which we will explore in the next section.

REFLECTION QUESTIONS

- Where do you see cultural appropriation in yoga?

- Do you see how addressing the causes of separation, such as cultural appropriation, are necessary for moving toward true unity and equity?

- Consider your position—is it one of power and privilege over the source culture and how might your relationship to yoga, such as profiting off it, mean you are causing harm?

YOGA AND GLAMORIZATION

As we continue to understand the way separation shows up in yoga in the West, we need to look at one facet of cultural appropriation called glamorization. Visiting a local studio can be a study in glamorization.

I recall walking through a casual beachside town that could have been many places in the West, on a day not long ago. I sauntered into a yoga studio shop: An *Om* symbol glinted off the outside wall, a bronze *Shiva* statue greeted me when I walked into the studio, tanks and t-shirts dangled on a rack shouting promises and threats—"But first, yoga," "What Up, Ommie," and "Namaslay"—above tight leggings. This is the normative representation of yoga today.

Glamorization involves taking cultural symbols, signs, art and iconography out of context and using them for one's own purposes to telegraph spirituality or wisdom (Deshpande, 2019).

Often, this type of glamorization is appropriation because the use of the sign or symbol bears little resemblance to the source culture from which it originated. And often the use of the symbols or iconography is, at best, odd or out of place, and, at worst, outright disrespectful to the source culture. Yoga is often used as a prop to create a certain aesthetic or "look." For instance, how yoga poses appear on Instagram, on magazine covers and marketing from predominantly able-bodied, pretty-privileged, white, cisgender (persons whose gender identity matches their biological sex at birth) women.

Orientalism is a key element in the practice of glamorization that has a long history in the interactions between the West and East.

Edward W. Said, in his thought-provoking book, *Orientalism*, defines it as having started during the enlightenment period of the 1600s and is the acceptance in the West of, "the basic distinction between East and West as the starting point for elaborate theories, epics, novels, social descriptions, and political accounts concerning the Orient, its people, customs, 'mind,' destiny and so on" (1979).

Glamorization is rooted in the orientalist way of seeing that exaggerates and distorts the differences of Asians and Asian culture. This orientalization is dangerous in that it is a stereotypical oversimplification and it often includes seeing Asians as backward, uncivilized, weak and dangerous.

Glamorization and stereotypes can be harmful because they are based on the superiority of one group over others, as well as stereotypes that diminish the dignity and worth of whole groups of people.

Virtue signaling is a form of glamorization.

Virtue signaling is a way of telegraphing your hipness by referencing any of our Indigenous / Black / Asian / Global South / Third-World cultures.

Words and phrases such as "guru," "spirit animal," "spiritual gangsta," "boho" or "tribe" constitute "virtue signaling," which can be thought of as "coolness by appropriation."

To be clear: I am not saying don't use Sanskrit language or practices inherent to the yoga tradition. Use them respectfully. Take time to build a relationship with them. Get to know them. And if possible, don't use them in ways that tokenize, objectify or cause harm.

An example of glamorization that causes harm is when a Western t-shirt company takes the image of *Ganesh* and puts it on a shirt with a blunt in one hand, a bottle of alcohol in another, a gun in another and a knife in another.

This causes harm in a number of ways. First, it is disrespectful to the many people who see and experience *Ganesh* as a representation of the divine.

Second, it is harmful because this non-Indian-owned t-shirt company is part of systemic imbalance of power, profiting off something that is not part of their culture by using it in an inappropriate way.

Another example of glamorization is adopting different cultural symbols that become forward-thinking, fashionable or cool when adopted by white people, but when an Indian person displays them are considered backward or traditionalist, at best, or a threat to society, at worst.

We see this most strikingly within the Sikh community, who wear turbans as part of their faith, but in the United States have been persecuted and even killed for wearing this marker of religious faith. White *kundalini*

practitioners can take on and off their turbans as a spiritual signifier with no or much less fear of being harmed.

Glamorization is one way that yoga culture gets exotified, glamorized and portioned-out in ways that disrespect part of the practice without bringing it together in a unified whole.

REFLECTION QUESTIONS

- Where do you specifically see glamorization in your own yoga space, studio, home practice space, within your yoga clothes or equipment?

- Are you using "*namaste*" as yoga lingo to create a certain vibe in your studio, or as a heartfelt greeting?

- Where could you connect to cultural stewards and lineage holders to learn more about the cultural elements, rituals and symbols of this practice?

YOGA AND STERILIZATION

Sterilization is another aspect of separation, causing cultural appropriation on the opposite extreme from glamorization. Both operate in a system of acquiring riches, knowledge or wealth from another culture and extracting from it for one's own gain without respecting the culture of origin.

The sterilization of yoga happens when the cultural meaning, history and practices are stripped away.

We see sterilization at work, for example, with "No-Om yoga," "No-ga," forbidding mantras and using Sanskrit words or phrases in ways that do not honor the practice.

For example, recently *Scientific American* (Andre, 2019) described *Anuloma Viloma*, otherwise known as alternate nostril breathing, a calming breathing technique where one breathes in and out through one nostril and then the other, with no reference to its historical practice as part of yogic *pranayama*, as Cardiac Coherence Breathing. This is the appropriation of yogic practices as seen through an orientalist, scientifically backed, white-supremacist fantasy.

Often, this practice of sterilization is justified by saying that the "dogma" needs to be removed so that it makes yoga more "accessible." This approach is problematic because it assumes that the practice as it was originally imagined and created isn't accessible in the first place, or that somehow now we (a white-centering, modernized normative perspective) know better.

In this view, the original Indian practitioners and stewards of yoga are seen as backward or uncivilized. By sterilizing the practice of its cultural overtones it becomes safe for white, normative consumption. This sterilization is not just benign. It is serving a larger white-supremacist agenda of making the practice less "foreign" and more palatable for the dominant white culture.

Note that the practice of sterilization is a tricky and complex issue. It can intersect with the use of skillful means. For example, there are times and places where a yoga teacher may bring in the Sanskrit terminology or philosophical elements of yoga slowly, such as when teaching two-to-five-year-olds. The teacher may do their best to use skillful means to share the full expanse of the practice. For example, I share yoga *asana* and speak about the yoga practice of kindness when I teach in my son's preschool. There is a difference between being skillful and attuned to the community one is connecting with and intentionally removing elements from the practice to make it more palatable to a normative audience.

HARM REDUCTION: IS IT POSSIBLE TO BE NON-INDIAN AND TEACH YOGA WITHOUT APPROPRIATING?

This is a tricky question.

In general, it is not entirely possible not to appropriate given our post-colonial cultural context, global capitalism, and the white supremacy and white centering within the West.

While we may not be able to completely eradicate appropriation, we can learn more, do far better and do less harm, which is what we are doing with the project of learning to honor and not appropriate. As we explore how to appropriate less, we need to keep close the ideas of progress and not perfection, as well as harm reduction.

Harm reduction aims at reducing harm, atoning for harm done and moving forward in ways that reduce the impact of harm on as many people as possible.

Keep in mind as we explore cultural appropriation that we are considering it within a context and that we are exploring the causes of separation. These will be addressed and solutions will be offered in the sections on Reconnection and Liberation.

REFLECTION QUESTIONS

- Where around you do you see sterilization in yoga and where have you sterilized yoga?

- How can you bring more of the complex fullness of the eightfold pillars of yoga into your study, learning and/or teaching?

- Do you think it is possible to reduce harm, practice or teach and appropriate less or without appropriating? How?

- If you would like resources to check yourself—and we should be checking ourselves all the time—get the Embrace Yoga Checklist at embraceyogaresources.com.

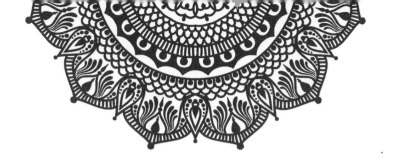

PART 3

YOGA CULTURE AND TRAUMA

"There's really no such thing as the 'voiceless'. There are only the deliberately silenced, or the preferably unheard."

— ARUNDHATI ROY

YOGIS AND TRAUMA

As we look closer at the causes of separation, it is important that we address the context from which yoga as a practice emerges. Trauma is embedded in many facets of our social systems and history and impacts yogic contexts, as well.

As we have explored, cultural appropriation happens in a context of power imbalance and harm. The context that yoga has come to us in the West itself is embedded with trauma.

As yogis in the West, it would benefit us individually, and the yoga community as a whole, to learn about and address trauma. Trauma is ubiquitous. It is present in most studios, schools and yoga classes. It is woven into the fabric of our society and the way we share or create space to teach or learn yoga today.

Trauma is anything overwhelming that impacts the nervous system in a way in which we are unable to cope or respond, as defined by Dr. Bessel van der Kolk (2017), a psychiatrist and researcher on post-traumatic stress. Trauma causes biological, physiological, emotional, mental and behavioral challenges. Trauma can be of multiple kinds: developmental trauma, shock trauma and trauma related to systemic injustice.

A YOGIC PERSPECTIVE ON TRAUMA: YOGA IS A SCIENCE OF TRAUMA HEALING

Yoga has always had a perspective of seeking to heal trauma and alleviate inner and outer anguish. From ancient times, some thousands of years ago, *rishis*, *yogis*, and *sanyasis* were involved in practices to find freedom from suffering. These teachings were passed down for thousands of years through oral tradition—word of mouth—from teacher to student. The primary aim was to seek liberation from the things that cause us suffering.

We will explore briefly some resources for further exploration and tools for coping with and handling trauma as they are key for supporting us as we address separation. It is beyond the scope of this book to elucidate the full scope of yogic practices to address trauma, but it is important to note that many yogic practices in the different systems of yoga—including *Patanjali's* eight limbs, *yamas, niyamas, asana, pranayama, pratyahara, dharana, dhyana* and *samadhi*, as well as other practices developed and codified by yogic practitioners such as *mantra* and *mudra*—offer complex and systematic methods to amplify calm and peace and reduce anxiety and trauma in the mind-body-spirit system.

YOGIS AND COLONIAL TRAUMA

S
E
P
A
R
A
T
I
O
N

I build on the work of Dr. Joy DeGruy, Resmaa Menakem, David Emerson, and others to postulate that there is another kind of trauma that particularly pertains to yoga culture and its context, called "colonial trauma."

Colonial trauma is a kind of systemic trauma where the colonial or post-colonial system seeks to divide and separate, control the resources (cultural, material, natural wealth) and exploit the resources of a target group, causing ongoing complex trauma (Barkataki, 2019).

The trauma of colonization can happen during colonization and post-colonization as the impacts of the erasure of culture, norms, behaviors and practices are intersectional and cumulative over time.

Institutional and systematic colonial violence, which seeks to control, deny and exploit, can lead to symptoms such as cultural dissynchrony (feeling out of place within one's culture), disorientation and feeling isolated, not at home in one's environment, out of sync with culture, time and place, a lack of purpose, and personal internalized oppression. Those impacted exhibit symptoms not unlike PTSD—hypervigilance, depression and personal and social anxiety. (Khouri, Hala. 2020)

This can show up in the bodies of BIPOC folks feeling disoriented, disconnected, having a sense of tightness and stress in the belly and chest, tension headaches and health concerns such as increased heart rate, high blood pressure and other forms of physical disease. It can show up mentally and emotionally through anxiety, depression, stress and other forms of psychological and emotional trauma.

This trauma impacts the mind, body and spirit, so yoga can be an effective tool for healing.

Entitlement to pick and choose and to take what we want from the yogic system because it benefits us without regard for those we are impacting is called "colonial supremacy."

We may see colonial trauma and colonial supremacy forces at play in yoga spaces today in the following ways:

- Characteristics of many/most Western yoga spaces: Cold, quiet, clean, bare
- Yoga culture can be filled with competition and specialization
- Expert status—a consolidation of knowledge and power
- Interactions are transactional and rigid

This contrasts with traditional yoga in the following ways that I observed in my travels and practice in North, Central and South India, as well as in my practice within Indian yogic communities in the diaspora. Instead of cold, quiet and bare spaces such as in the West, in traditional yoga teachings often happen in community and collectivized spaces. It is quite common for yogis to be seen in connection and conversation in community. For example, instead of a focus on competition and individualism, traditional yoga encourages a humility, respect for teachers and traditions and a lack of focus on the self. Instead of simply focusing on expert status, there is an understanding that knowledge resides in the *Vedas*, the sacred texts, as well as many divine and inspired teachers. Traditionally, interactions are not transactional but rather embedded in relationship.

Colonial trauma leads modern yogis in the West to perpetuate dehumanization. Just as early colonialism sought to divide and separate, control, deny and exploit.

The antidote is connection and unification, uplifting and belonging to one another. Often the community-care models that are most effective today for dealing with trauma are similar to the collectivized, non-hierarchical community and collective living spaces of many indigenous ancestors.

Part of the work of reclaiming the roots of yoga is living and practicing yoga as a way of being, a philosophy and way of life. We invite this in by asking: Do my choices lead to more separation or more unity?

Indigenous and traditional practices of mutuality can help to rebuild cultural rhythms. These include storytelling; listening to the stories of past trials and challenges builds resilience. Engaging in ritual and rites of passage. Practicing nonattachment—*swaraj*—connecting to our *karma* and taking personal responsibility while working toward our *dharma* or purpose. Opening to understand a more cyclical nature of time and healing.

Though colonial trauma is pervasive, fractures culture and creates disorientation and separation, yoga is a way of being, a philosophy and way of life, and its deep practice leads to unity.

With the practice of yoga, we can experience holistic recovery, self-control and personal responsibility that allows disorientation to transform into integration and connection.

WHY DOES COLONIAL TRAUMA MATTER TODAY?

Trauma treatment and recovery is embedded deep within yoga practice and philosophy as well as in yoga's sister science, *Ayurveda*, though the discussion of this is beyond the scope of this book.

However, looking at the ways indigenous Indians have processed and held space for trauma is an important part of reclaiming these traditions.

What I've observed is that colonial trauma impacts everything from the way yoga was passed from teacher to student to how and why it came to the West, to the kinds of spaces we create today. Colonial trauma, race-based trauma and its corollary, white supremacy, are all part of cultural appropriation and other systems of separation at play in yoga today. In order to heal and transform, we need to understand the systems in which we are participating.

Colonial trauma is specific and an important issue to address in yoga culture. When we are engaging trauma, we must consider the roots of that trauma so we don't perpetuate cycles of harm.

This work is on colonial and post-colonial trauma and its impacts in our context today, as well as how we can personally and collectively heal these traumas rather than repeat them.

REFLECTION QUESTIONS

How was yoga passed on to you or your yoga instructor/teacher?

What supplemental reading will you do on colonial trauma?

I named some examples above. Where do **you** see systemic and colonial trauma embedded within the context of your experience of yoga today?

TRAUMA-INFORMED YOGA RESOURCES

"I do not view post-traumatic stress disorder as a pathology to be managed, suppressed or adjusted to, but the result of a natural process gone awry. Healing trauma requires direct experience of the living, feeling, knowing organism."

—PETER LEVINE, PH.D.

As we begin to explore trauma-informed yoga, please note that this does not take the place of speaking to your doctor or a credentialed mental health professional. Also, consider that trauma and healing have been a part of yogic and *Ayurvedic* science for thousands of years. We are developing practices and study in the West to name and speak to things that have been practiced for a long time.

My understanding of trauma-informed yoga as part of the roots of yoga is influenced by many teachers at Kerala Ayurveda, as well as Shankarji, Kabir, Dr. Shaila Vaidya, Candace Martin and Hala Khouri as well as others in the field.

If **trauma** is anything overwhelming that impacts the nervous system in a way in which we are unable to cope or respond and causes fragmentation, then addressing trauma is accomplished by bringing harmony and integration.

As taught by trauma researcher Peter Levine, Ph.D., in addressing trauma, it is helpful to develop and sustain a **resource**.

According to David Emerson (2015), a resource is anything that creates a sense of internal safety, enabling us to explore, unpack and make sense of a past experience. Uniting with a resource can feel empowering. It connects us to the feeling of control within.

He and other researchers in modern neurobiology of trauma find that these systems of yogic practice address all the levels of fragmentation and disorientation in the brain to try to bring wholeness and healing.

S
E
P
A
R
A
T
I
O
N

Our heritage and resources from the yoga tradition are often supported by modern neuroscience. We have multiple parts of our brains that address different needs and functions. Ancient systems for healing have been studied and seen to address these different functionalities.

TRAUMA-INFORMED YOGA IN THE CONTEXT OF INDIAN YOGA HISTORY

Yogic teachings were passed down for thousands of years through oral tradition, from teacher to student. The main aim was seeking liberation from the things that cause us suffering and include a direct description of what it means to be trauma-informed and spiritually aware.

We can find specific practices to address trauma in the earliest Vedic yoga texts.

One of the main teachings is *Tat Tvam Asi*—"you art that"—from the Chandogya Upanishad 6.8.7 of the *Sama Veda*.

Practically speaking, what this means to us in our own experience is that we, as the local point of consciousness, are not separate or different from Universal Consciousness. Just as we are all the same as the Universal, you and I are also not separate or different in our innermost being. We are having this experience in the depth of yoga or meditative absorption, immersed in the unity of just being.

The understanding of yoga as unity can also invite us to bring this alive in our day-to-day lives. From meditation or practice on our mat to welcoming people into our studios and classrooms, we can practice yoga as transformation of trauma, yoga as healing and unity.

CHANTING MANTRA SUCH AS AUM

As B.K.S. Iyengar (1979) elucidates in *Light on Yoga*, the sacred sound

Aum addresses the three aspects of existence, and he shares this experiential practice.

1. "Ah": From base of spine to navel (creation)—correlates to the brain stem
2. "Uu": Navel to throat, sustaining (that which pervades)—correlates to the limbic system
3. "Mm": Throat to crown (transform); that which transforms and transcends—correlates to the neocortex

The entire sound together creates a unitive, whole, harmonized brain.

AYURVEDA CAN BE SEEN AS A FRAMEWORK FOR HEALING FROM TRAUMA.

Ayurveda comes from *ayuh* meaning "life" or "longevity" and *veda* meaning "study of." Therefore, *Ayurveda* is the study of life.

Ayurvedic practitioners understand the five elements of earth, water, fire, air and ether (space) are the five elements that make up all that exists in our universe. Each one of us has a unique mind and body constitution made up of these elements combined to make our own *Ayurvedic* fingerprint. This distinctive constitution is called our *prakriti*, or mind-body type. Some people colloquially call our unique type our *dosha*.

The *doshas* are made up of the five elements and are called *vata*, *pitta*, and *kapha*.

Kapha is conceived of the elements earth and water and correlates to the emotions of depression.

Pitta is conceived of the elements fire and water and correlates to the emotions of anger.

Vata is conceived of the elements air and space and correlates to anxiety and that which moves.

Knowing this, *Ayurvedic* trauma-aware recommendations for harmonizing and balancing the *doshas* can help identify our coping mechanisms and address trauma in the moment and over time.

S
E
P
A
R
A
T
I
O
N

HARMONIZING

Ayurvedically, we are taught to rebalance by harmonizing with nature and one's surroundings.

The five senses can be a wonderful way to harmonize. As we mobilize head, neck and shoulders we release stress and have an immediate sense of being in present time. Turning the head can cue the parasympathetic nervous system to come online. One practice that many different trainers and therapists use and that teachers of mindfulness share is to do a countdown and notice: five things you hear, four things you see, three things you can touch/feel, two things you can smell and one thing you can taste.

GROUNDING/ANCHORING/ROOTING

According to trauma researcher Emerson (2015), when we feel threatened (whether the threat is real or perceived), we may feel groundless. We can begin to pay attention to all the places that touch a supporting surface. We can notice where our physical bodies meet the earth, chair, mat or floor to help create a feeling of support and strength.

SELF-RULE—CENTERING

"Heart/Belly/Breath"

The yogic concept of *swaraj*, or self-rule, helps us locate our center of power within ourselves. We can explore inner awareness around the heart or belly to find internal guidance. When we are able to, checking in with sensation helps us re-center ourselves. It enables us to feel, find and move from a place of expansive inner power and choice (Barkataki, Wardha, 2007).

BREATHING/PRANAYAMA

Breathing practices along with their benefits have been described in early yogic texts. Now, scientific research has shown breathing can help harmonize the autonomic nervous system and lower your heart rate. Breathing is a process that is both automatic and self-regulated. How we breathe has an impact on our physiology. Traditionally, counting breath and keeping inhales and exhales equal or taking longer exhales moves us into a more calm state.

SYSTEMATIC RELAXATION/YOGA NIDRA

This involves using the techniques of systematic relaxation central to the yogic tradition. Whether used to give the practitioner some space from the uncomfortable human body or to help put the practitioner to sleep, the practice of relaxation is helpful. *Yoga nidra* and other practices of deep relaxation have been shown to decrease anxiety, reprogram addictions and lead participants to greater wellbeing.

MEDITATION

This is a process of focusing the mind. It is a multifaceted practice. Sitting meditation involves sitting in one spot and focusing the mind on a particular object of focus such as following the breath. Walking meditation using steps and movement in alignment with *mantra* or the breath is good when you need to release energy or are feeling anxious. Meditation can be a helpful practice for checking in and resourcing ourselves. *Metta* meditation, or loving kindness meditation, can be practiced to help handle trauma as well.

ASANAS FOR ANXIETY

Practicing specific yoga *asana* in a slow fashion, close to the earth, can be very grounding and soothing. For example:

Windmill arms, Shaking the body—getting wiggles out.
Tadagasana (Pond Shape)
Balasana (Child's Shape)
Urdhva Mukha Svanasana (Upward-Facing Dog Shape)

Simhasana (Lion's Shape)

Viparita Karani (Sleeping Tiger or Legs Up the Wall)

Specifically using "shape" or "form" or "expression" instead of pose is a way to move us in the West away from thinking yoga is just something we do rather than something we express and are.

SELF-CARE AND SELF-KEEPING

This is a practice of self-love and healing. Placing your hand on your own heart to share love and comfort with yourself. Practice *abhyanga* (oil massage). Be in nature, perhaps go to the beach, sit under a large tree, or practice gardening. Engage a gratitude practice and journal writing.

CONNECTION AND COMMUNITY CARE

As we heal from trauma it can be helpful to find ourselves in community. Volunteer. Spend time with animals. Reach out and share with supportive friends. Connect.

Now that we have addressed some tools to help us deal with the trauma and challenges of separation, we will continue on our examination of these challenges in order to achieve unity.

REFLECTION QUESTIONS

❀ What are some key elements of a yogic perspective on trauma that stand out to you?

❀ Where can you see the indigenous Indian roots of trauma-informed yoga within the yoga tradition?

❀ Which supportive tools or resources will you try in your community?

YOGIS AND ADDRESSING SYSTEMIC TRAUMA

Trauma builds up over time from dealing with interlocking systems of oppression: sexism, racism, ableism, heterosexism, transphobia, classism or other systemic injustices (Menakem, 2017).

For example, the impact of race, gender or sexuality-based violence, institutional and systemic racism, sexism, white supremacy / white dominance, homophobia and heteronormativity can lead to symptoms not unlike PTSD—hypervigilance, depression and anxiety. Trauma can become cumulative.

Colonization and post-colonization are examples of systemic trauma. Colonization is taking power away from some while those in a position of power benefit from the exploitation of natural resources, labor, the soul, spirit or ideas of indigenous people and their cultural knowledge. Colonizing yoga is not just a metaphor—it's a practice that continues in an unequal relationship of exploitation.

As we will address, colonization is a system, not a one-time event, and it can have ongoing repercussions and impacts. It is also a re-traumatization.

For example, I have experienced the impacts of colonial trauma within my own family.

I visited my Bengali and Assamese (Northeast Indian) family recently. I'd been delving deep into yoga's roots and inquiring about the culture from which yoga emerged.

Excited to learn more directly, I asked my own father and aunts about our culture's history. I was excited to hear their educated perspective of our own Indian culture and the great civilizations from which we are descended.

I prompted, "Tell me what you learned in school about the Indus River Valley Civilization and the culture that yoga emerged from."

What they said in response floored me.

They looked at me. My father said, "I can tell you about the British battles of Culloden and Blenheim."

My aunt, who lives in Kolkata, a city rich in Indian culture and history, added, "I can tell you many of the British empire's accomplishments but nothing much about India before British empire."

"But, wait," I said, forgetting good manners in my shock. "You aren't *that* old. You went to school *after* India gained independence from the British. Why don't you know about our cultural accomplishments? About *our* history?"

"That's what our schools taught," my aunt replied. They both shrugged.

Imagine my incredulous shock. Indian citizens in a *free* India learned from Indian teachers about the British empire and not their own history?

What kept running through my mind was this question: *How many years does it take to erase thousands of years of civilization?*

This is happening right here and right now. Colonization exists in the lasting legacy of empire on the forgotten histories of a colonized people. The erasure of thousands of years of profound cultural advancements, philosophical training and social developments.

This is what we mean when we talk about the colonization of yoga now.

Without knowing it, when we roll out our mats we may just be scratching the surface of what it means to practice yoga. We are, intentionally or unintentionally, enacting an erasure, a forgetting.

We say and feel that yoga is union. But can a practice interwoven with division lead us to union? And if so, how can it?

The colonization of India and its cultural gifts, traditions and spirituality such as yoga has an impact on us *now*. How can Western teachers and students of yoga move forward honoring their own journey as well as embracing yoga's roots? How can we begin to practice yoga as union today?

A first step is working to deepen our understanding and practice of yoga, taking its colonial history into consideration. I share this exploration with the spirit of love and appreciation for you. Wherever you are from. You are part of me. I am part of you. We all have ancestors. We all have history and culture. And we all matter.

I don't want you to stop teaching or practicing yoga. I want you to understand and know its context is relevant for us today.

For many yogis today, we are either experiencing, moving through, perpetuating or healing systemic trauma.

It's important that if you're a teacher who does not hold a marginalized racialized identity, you become culturally competent enough to be intentional with your language in classes you teach. In response to others' concerns, saying things such as, "That's not what I experience," or, "Maybe that's just a story you're creating," is hurtful and can perpetuate and even cause trauma.

With the tool of yoga as teacher, we can lessen the harm of traumas that we may not be aware we have been perpetuating. Yoga itself can be our guide in this practice of unpacking harm and increasing personal and global empathy.

REFLECTION QUESTIONS

⚙ Brainstorm some examples of how many yoga spaces in the West replicate systems of harm and create trauma for many non-normative people.

⚙ Check in with your own mind-body-spirit system as we address trauma. Where are you holding tension in your body? Can you breathe there?

⚙ What practices may help you in releasing this tension or trauma?

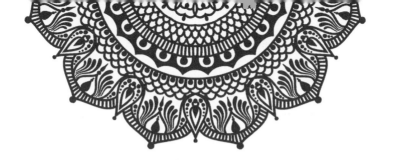

PART 4

YOGA NORMS, OPPRESSION AND WHITE SUPREMACY

*"I'm for truth, no matter who tells it. I'm for justice,
no matter who it is for or against. I'm a human being, first
and foremost, and as such I'm for whoever and whatever
benefits humanity as a whole."*

— MALCOLM X

YOGIS AND OPPRESSION

The harm of cultural appropriation of yoga is directly tied to systemic oppression, so let's explore what that is. Our exploration of oppression and white supremacy is a direct way to practice *satya*, or truth-telling and exploration.

S
E
P
A
R
A
T
I
O
N

Systemic oppression is the political, economic, social and cultural putting-down of people, groups or individuals.

Oppression lifts some up at the expense of pushing others down. Oppression is also about who holds power and how they wield that power.

It is important to note that "reverse racism" isn't possible in a system that holds up, privileges and benefits one group, namely white people, at the expense of all others.

It is systemic, institutional power that has come to be historically and continues over time. Oppression allows certain "groups" of people to assume a dominant position over other "groups" and this dominance is maintained at an institutional level.

INTERNALIZED OPPRESSION

A powerful realization here is that oppression can also be internalized. That happens when someone from a target group takes in discriminatory beliefs about themselves. This has huge implications for self-esteem and success in life.

Systems of oppression run through our language and shape the way we act and do things in our culture, including in social institutions and yoga culture.

A social institution is a system created by human beings that often has great power in society. Yoga has become a social institution in the West, carrying with it its own norms.

SOCIAL/CULTURAL NORMS

Systems of oppression are built around what are understood to be "norms" in our societies. A norm signifies what is "normal," acceptable, desirable. "The norm" is something that is valued in a society. Yoga too has its own norms. And they are quite evident. When we begin to look directly at them we can see more of what needs to be transformed.

For example, a system of oppression that impacts us is the idea that certain bodies are "normal" while other bodies are abnormal, such as bigger bodies or people with disabilities. This is deeply harmful psychologically and is perpetuated in the yoga industry both explicitly and unconsciously.

REFLECTION QUESTIONS

⚛ Think about a time you realized that yoga had a "look." What are some "norms" in yoga culture in the West?

⚛ How and where do you fit the norm? How and where do you deviate from it? How does it feel in both cases?

⚛ How may norms surrounding yoga in the West be connected to systems bigger than ourselves—that is to say, to the systems of oppression?

S
E
P
A
R
A
T
I
O
N

YOGIS AND WHITE SUPREMACY

Norms in yoga in the West are directly tied to a system of oppression called white supremacy.

White supremacy is the belief that white people are superior to all other races and that they should therefore hold the highest positions in society and dominate other races (hooks, 2018).

White supremacists differ from white supremacy. White supremacists are individuals dedicated to racial nationalism and who want to grow a white-dominant nation-state. White supremacy is a system that privileges one group over all others.

The issue is, white supremacy encompasses beliefs that often are unconscious, implicit biases. This is important to note: Frequently people get caught in white exceptionalism, such as thinking, "I don't believe white people are superior therefore white supremacy doesn't apply to me."

It is also important not to get caught in trying to prove "I'm not a bad person," or "I'm not a racist." This is actually beside the point. Racism and white supremacy are all around us, one individual's interactions with it notwithstanding.

According to theorist bell hooks, white supremacy is like the air we breathe. It's the default in our society. Our yoga context in the West is an integral part of society. If we look closely, the yoga context in the West, in many ways, glorifies white normativity and white supremacy far more than other sectors, like sports, education and, increasingly, politics.

WHY TALK ABOUT WHITE SUPREMACY AND YOGA?

If we want to change or stop participating in systems that are causing harm, we need to understand what the systems are. White supremacy is a critical part of yoga culture. For you, it may be internalized, it may be underground, but it is likely there. When we examine it, we can address it, rather than perpetuate it.

We say yoga, *yuj*, is unity.

But there are blocks to unity, which means harm is done. Unity doesn't mean erasing or ignoring someone's reality or lived experience simply for the sake of "being one" or staying "positive." Here, we mean uniting our humanity while understanding the many systems that oppress *specific* people and protect other *specific* people. Oppression *is* the separation that the practice is inviting us to heal.

Keep in mind that by identifying white supremacy culture we are not attempting to cancel culture for all white people. White supremacy culture is a powerful norm tied to oppression and colonization, and harms all of us. With this in mind let's examine this culture in yoga.

WHITE SUPREMACY CULTURE IN YOGA

White supremacy culture in yoga looks like a focus on the following:
- Perfectionism
- Singularity and individualism
- Lack of diversity
- Yoga norms controlled by a single narrative and single representation
- Exclusion of, policing and shaming of anything that differs from the norm, i.e. Brown, fat or less-able bodies
- Focus on physical attainment and worship of the physical body

Yoga today has a white supremacy culture problem.

My understanding of this is informed by experts in the field of culture such as the piece "White Supremacy Culture" by Tema Okun and Kenneth Jones (2001).

In preparation for writing this book, I scrolled through #yoga on Instagram and saw how deeply problematic this single narrative is. Image after image of people who don't look like me or my Indian ancestors were in various degrees of acrobatic yoga poses. This didn't look anything like the yoga that I had been taught by my family or teachers in India. In fact, the dominant narrative looks like the pages of a conventional magazine. *For*

a practice meant to be freeing, why are the images so confining? I had to ask myself.

We are here together to challenge yoga's white supremacy culture.

Reflect on what and where you see white supremacy culture in yoga, especially in your own life and around you. It is particularly insidious in how we talk to ourselves about our own bodies and our own practice.

Consider how you might change white supremacy culture to something else.

For example, here are some anti-white-supremacy Embrace Yoga Commitments:

- Instead of taking an individualistic approach, highlight community.
- Instead of focusing on perfecting postures, focus on the process of feeling a yoga *asana* shape express itself in an individual's unique body.
- Offer yourself and others incremental growth that supports where someone is.
- Instead of yoga celebrities, create and uplift communities.
- Instead of obsession with the body, focus on obsession with the heart, service, intuition and spiritual realization and freedom.
- Instead of frontlining more white yoga teachers, or tokenizing BIPOC, invite, uplift and provide platforms for multiple teachers of color in every yoga space.
- Instead of solely focusing on physicality and aesthetics of how yoga looks, focus on yoga philosophy, ethics and spirituality.

To get to unity we can't simply ignore the things that cause separation. White supremacy comes from separation, so we must explore and understand the tools of separation. We need to see, look at and bring the things that separate us to light so we can address them. Dismantle them. Build toward true unity with the real tools of yoga to embrace yoga.

REFLECTION QUESTIONS

- Where do you see white supremacy culture in yoga spaces and yoga culture in the West?

- Where in your studios or communities, in-person or online, is white supremacy culture being interrupted and different models upheld or shown?

- What are your anti-white-supremacy commitments to embrace yoga's roots?

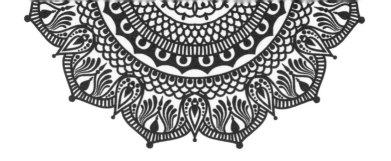

PART 5

YOGIS AND THE TOOLS OF SEPARATION

"I believe that virtually all the problems in the world come from inequality of one kind or another."

—Amartya Sen

YOGIS AND RACISM

Race is a social construct that classifies human beings as a more or less distinct group because of shared physical traits such as skin color. Though race is a social construct, the impact and harm that occurs based on race is all too real.

In *Why are All the Black Kids Sitting Together in the Cafeteria* (Tatum 1998), racism is defined as any attitude, action, or practice backed up by institutional power that harms people because they belong to a particular racial group; a system of social, economic, political, or other advantage/ privilege bestowed on people who possess certain physical traits. It is often described as *prejudice + power*—a phrase Patricia Bidol coined in the 1970s. This definition has been used and elaborated on by psychologist Beverly Tatum (Ibid.) and others working in anti-racism.

Prejudice is a pre-judgment about someone or something based on assumptions. The acting-out of prejudice in a way that harms a person or group is discrimination.

YOGIS AND MICROAGGRESSIONS

Microaggressions are everyday actions, slights, indignities, put-downs and insults that target populations (BIPOC, women, LGBTQ+ people) experience in their day-to-day lives. Microaggressions are a part of a system of inequity and add up for those who are the target of them (PBS, 2006).

Many microaggressions occur in yoga spaces. Indian colleagues often mention how many times someone has commented on how "exotic" they look, or asked them the correct way to pronounce a Sanskrit word. My colleagues of size comment how often they get looked up and down or side-eyed in a yoga class. The same goes for people of color, older folks, gender non-conforming or trans folks or those with disabilities. Microaggressions may not register to the aggressor as an act of racism, transphobia, exclusion or aggression, but they are.

Many marginalized people and BIPOC don't accept the term 'microaggression' because the harm done doesn't feel 'micro,' but large.

Here are some examples of microaggressions common in Western yoga spaces:

- Making fun of someone's first or last name or its pronunciation
- Saying, "You do this so well," or "You're so good at this," or "Wow, you say that so well."
- Asking a bigger-bodied practitioner if they are sure they can handle the class

- Asking a person of color if they work at the studio
- Telling a teacher of color they are the first POC teacher they've ever had

YOGIS AND IMPLICIT AND EXPLICIT BIAS

Implicit bias is a prejudice toward a person or group of people that turns into an action unconsciously.

My colleague, a Black man, walked into a typical yoga class. Upon doing so, he found that some of the students grasped their belongings closer to themselves. Some even moved to separate areas of the room from where he was practicing.

The students may not be aware they are acting out their bias, but they are exhibiting implicit bias and that bias causes harm.

Explicit bias is the conscious acting-out or behavior based on a prejudice toward a person or group of people. For example, when a student moves their position because they didn't want to practice next to a man of color, that is discrimination.

These actions of implicit and explicit bias carry immense harm by making the person feel unworthy, dismissed and unwelcome in the space.

An important note is that we often struggle to see the microaggressions that we ourselves perpetuate. It becomes even more crucial to practice *svadhyaya* and self-reflect.

The impact of implicit and explicit bias is still the same, so it doesn't necessarily matter if you meant to cause harm or not. If harm was done, it must be addressed. The first step to addressing harm is to acknowledge it. Next, apologize and atone for the harm caused and learn more to prevent future harm. Finally, start to work toward equity and uplifting others.

REFLECTION QUESTIONS

◉ In yoga spaces, what microaggressions or implicit and explicit bias have you seen, overheard, experienced or contributed to?

◉ How can you begin or contribute to creating an environment where microaggressions, implicit and explicit bias are not perpetrated?

◉ How can we combat racism using yoga?

"Yoga world, if you are tired of hearing about colonization, racism and erasure, think for a breath about how tired some of us are experiencing it."

—Susanna Barkataki

YOGIS AND "I DON'T SEE COLOR"

"But aren't you causing more separation by talking about race? I don't see color. I see our souls. And your soul is beautiful. Everyone is equal." These are phrases I hear weekly.

"I don't see color," and its close cousins, "We are all one," "You are no different from me," "Stop being divisive," "That's reverse racism," and one that many BIPOC continue to hear in our industry, "But yoga means unity; let's just all be our divine nature together."

These phrases are micro or macro aggressions and all perpetuate the oppressive status quo while subtly or not-so-subtly gaslighting the person raising the question or concern. By gaslighting I mean undermining the beliefs and authority of the person who feels or sees prejudice.

From now forward, let's make sure the phrase "But we are all one—I don't see color," raises a red flag for people doing this work. The underlying belief is one that sees only individual experience and erases systemic injustice and differences.

Though this sentiment is beautiful, it erases the real material differences between BIPOC and those with white privilege.

The following are underlying beliefs behind the statement, "We are all one":

- I don't want to acknowledge the suffering or pain you might be in.
- I don't want to do the work to explore how I might be tacitly or overtly racist.
- I don't want you to think I'm racist, therefore this is all about me.
- I don't want to acknowledge that the world gives me privilege over you.
- I don't value your uniqueness as an individual and wish to bypass the reality that society treats you differently than it treats me.
- I can't be bothered to examine my biases, so I'm going to pretend I don't have any.

It can be hard to realize how we may have caused harm without even meaning to.

Yoga philosophy does see us as all connected, but not in a way that erases our different life experiences, challenges and the institutionalized and systemic oppressions that prevent us from accessing the same levels of growth, actualization and oneness.

To get to true oneness, we have to face the ways we may have been complicit in causing separation.

What you might say, to connect, instead of "I don't see color" is "I wonder how different your life experience might have been from mine. Can you tell me about it?"

In my own life, I have often found that when I open up and share the challenges of being treated as an "other" all through my childhood, it helps people understand that the sentiment of "we are all one" simply doesn't apply to some people.

However, it takes a lot of fortitude to share my own pain in order to educate someone about racial injustice. As a community we can move toward holding space for one another.

Rather than simply deny someone else's experience or pain, can we practice the art of holding tension and staying with the discomfort in a way that means we don't erase difference? This can be the art of holding anger, sadness, grief, betrayal or other challenging emotions that arise when we realize the world is not fair.

We can listen, hear another's experience, validate and care for their pain as well as work to create a world where this type of separation no longer exists.

REFLECTION QUESTIONS

◉ Why is saying, "I don't see color," and, "But we are all one," harmful or problematic?

◉ How do yoga spaces in the West perpetuate racism and what underlying false beliefs are at work in these spaces or within yourself that you can examine?

◉ What might you, or these institutions, teachers and companies do instead?

ERASURE, YOGA AND RACE: ON YOGA ORIGINS, SOUTH ASIANS AND APPROPRIATE ATTRIBUTION

Another misunderstanding is when people say, "Race isn't real." Though race is a construct it is violently real and has powerful impacts on lives. Correct naming is important. Racial categories are something we humans made up. But the discrimination that impacts someone based on race is not a fictitious thing, but incredibly harmful.

In the yoga industry, people are confused about what race or culture from which yoga comes. All too often people refer to yoga as coming from Southeast Asia or to me as Southeast Asian. But I'm not Southeast Asian.

This plays into the racist trope that all Asians look the same and are the same. This shows that people don't care enough or understand the rich and immense nuances among the different countries and cultures of Asia.

Asians have a vast array of cultures, practices, religions, foods and customs.

It is important to name us and our cultures correctly when you utilize practices, such as yoga, Tai Chi, Feng Shui or *Ayurveda*, to name a few, when referring to us and these practices.

Let's break it down. South Asians are from Afghanistan, Pakistan, India, Bangladesh, Nepal, Bhutan, Sri Lanka or Maldives.

East Asians are from China, Korea, Japan, Taiwan, Tibet or Mongolia.

Southeast Asians come from countries that are south of China, east of India. This includes eleven countries: Thailand, Vietnam, Malaysia, Singapore, the Philippines, Laos, Indonesia, Brunei, Burma (Myanmar), Cambodia and East Timor.

If you are talking about, practicing or using elements of our cultures and customs, it is respectful that you name and attribute us correctly. Please learn, understand and put this into practice.

Just as it is important to know this when referring to yoga, it's important to understand the difference between race and ethnicity.

Race refers to someone's skin color—melanin—and people are oppressed for the darkness of their skin. Ethnicity is a social group that has a common national or cultural tradition based on where they or their ancestry grew up. It's important to know the difference because an immigrant may be of a certain ethnicity, but will benefit from their proximity to whiteness due to white supremacy. Colorism is also a part of internalized and systemic oppression. For instance, someone may be privileged over another due to their whiteness.

Yoga has been used for oppressive purposes to exclude, hold down or oppress Dalits, Adivasis, and those who don't fit the religious majority in India. This too is misuse of yoga and is oppression and needs to be addressed.

YOGIS AND MISREPRESENTATION

South Asians and Desis (*Desis* is a term for diasporic Indians who live outside India) are actively excluded from positions of leadership in yoga.

The power structure works in such a way that when you exclude those from whom the teachings came, it makes it easier to erase us, then take a position where it is easy to steal and exploit this indigenous wisdom.

When you exclude folks from whom this medicine came, it further perpetuates exploitation and colonization in a global marketplace.

This also perpetuates the misrepresentation and watering-down of yoga.

There are many who don't speak up, but who experience similar displacement and even exclusion from yoga spaces.

YOGIS AND INVISIBILITY

When there are "white spaces missing faces," as Catrice M. Jackson aptly states in her book by that title—and in particular those that are Brown, disabled, queer, trans, bigger-bodied, disabled or otherwise marginalized people—irreparable harm is done.

YOGIS, MISREPRESENTATION AND BEING SEEN

If you were to do an image search for "yoga" right now you'd likely see what I mean. A sea of thin, white, cis-gendered women grace the screen. This is true in yoga magazines and in most mainstream yoga outlets in the West.

Consider that this practice was created, codified, developed and taught by Brown people for thousands of years.

Erasure of folks of color in yoga culture is painful. It happens continuously. If we take *Yoga Journal* covers as an example, we can see examples of erasure continuing.

Over the last 10 years, people of color have been on the cover less than a handful of times. Finally, when folks of color were on the cover, it coincided with the covers being split and half the cover in each case being given to white people, as well.

Nonrepresentation is part of a system of exclusion. No one intended to do it. In fact, most people involved in the *Yoga Journal* covers, as well as other organizations, media, schools and studios may be well-intentioned. But harm is still caused. Impact is always greater than intention.

Representation is important not only for equality and fairness, but also because it's a healing justice issue. When you don't see yourself represented in wellness and yoga spaces, it's hard to believe they are for you.

Though South Asian culture is one of the major places where the practice of yoga came from, was developed and cultivated and where yoga is still thriving, alive and well, South Asians are almost entirely erased from representation in yoga in the West.

This exclusion makes our indigenous knowledge and cultural wisdom that much easier to exploit. This unintentional exploitation is why reflecting and learning, as we will continue to do in the next section, is so key to embracing yoga.

REFLECTION QUESTIONS

⚙ Did you know the difference between South Asian and Southeast Asian? Why might this be important?

⚙ What new clarity do you now have about the importance of foregrounding South Asian yoga practitioners and teachers?

⚙ How as a yoga community can we do a better job of practicing inclusion and representation?

S
E
P
A
R

IV
REFLECTION

"Another world is not only possible, she is on her way.
On a quiet day, I can hear her breathing."

—Arundhati Roy

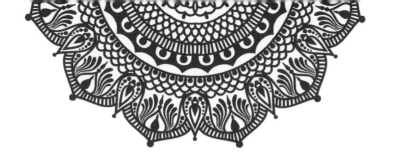

PART 1

PRIVILEGE, POWER, AND CULTURE

"Power is everywhere and comes from every where. In fact power produces; it produces reality; it produces domains of objects and rituals of truth."

—Michel Foucault

YOGIS AND THREE TYPES OF POWER

In this reflection section we start with assessing our own power that we hold, learn how we can cultivate it and use it wisely.

Yoga is a path toward unity and the practice itself cultivates power. As we do the work of reflecting on the causes of separation and go deeper into reflection on our role and how to embrace yoga's roots, it is necessary to look at power, what it is and how to use it. Once we understand and clarify our role in positions of power, we have tools to reduce harm in spaces and achieve justice and equity. Eventually, we can achieve unity.

Power is the ability to affect one's will on the world and create change.

According to the sociological work of Riane Eisler, there are three kinds of power. In order to embrace yoga, it is helpful to understand this framework of how power works.

First, there is "power over." Having power over someone is external power to control, dominate or enact one's will over another.

Next, there is "power with." Power with is power used for uplifting, supporting or helping another person.

Finally, there is "power within." Power within is internal power. This is a power that cannot be given or taken away. It is this kind of power that yoga cultivates (Eisler, 2007).

We also need to look at how power interacts directly with both violence and nonviolence.

The United States Institute of Peace and Center for Common Peace defines violence as any use of force that takes away the dignity or worth of another. They define nonviolence, or upstanding, as actions that protect, help or benefit the dignity and worth of another (Common Peace, 2004).

Power itself is neutral. It is a natural force. But power used violently or nonviolently directly changes the nature of that power. Let's examine the differences.

POWER OVER AND VIOLENCE

In modern history, colonizing powers, such as the British, used "power over" to take over the land of colonies then utilize and exploit the labor, natural resources, industrial power and anything deemed of value in that place.

We can see the misuse of "power over" founded in colonization continue into the modern day. Groups in positions of power colonize not only material resources, but also cultural riches. Now we have both colonization of land, or only physical resources, and we have colonization of cultural informational wealth, such as we see with yoga. Those in the West still have more power, wealth, access, etc.

A tangible example is a large US- or UK-based company that manufactures yoga leggings with deities on them. They benefit from the power imbalance that exists between India and the West.

Another example is the use of the white sage plant, taken from Native Americans and exploited by white people for profit and overharvested to the point of endangerment. In addition, this exploitation takes a spiritual practice, disconnects it from its original intention and gentrifies it.

Kory Snache (Giniw), an Anishinaabe from Chippewas of Rama Mnjiknini First Nation, says, "People who utilize sage spiritually have a very different concept of what sage is, and that should be respected." Kory continues, saying "It is deep-rooted with medicinal and spiritual understandings that are reinforced with teachings passed down through generations."

Usually this systemic imbalance of power involves exploitation. It can include the power to pick and choose what we take from a culture and to leave the rest behind without regard for the impact on the communities affected.

There are many ways that yoga spaces and yogis today use their power over others.

For example, as mentioned above, often sage-smudging is done prior to yoga class and passed off as traditional to yoga. Malas are used as a fashion trend rather than part of meditation practice. The *Om* symbol is used to telegraph spirituality, while those who wear it do not practice the unity it connotes.

REFLECTION

REFLECTION QUESTIONS

- Think of some examples of power over in yoga spaces or yoga communities today. Describe them.

- Where do you feel power in your life?

- Where do you feel you lack power?

- What, specifically, can/do you do to cultivate a healthy relationship with power?

YOGIS AND NONVIOLENT POWER

Just as power can be used violently, it can also be used nonviolently. This is the heart of yogic practice and the meaning of the first of *Patanjali's* ethical precepts laid out for yoga practitioners—*ahimsa* (non-harming or nonviolence).

In the Indian tradition, great effort and thought has been put into cultivating the practice of nonviolence. From the early works and explorations of Siddhartha Gautama, known as the Buddha, to Ashoka, the great emperor who wanted to share this path of nonviolence with the world, to the way India threw off the oppression of the British, studies in nonviolent power have shaped Indian history.

The yogic practice *of ahimsa* is not just the opposite of violence or about passively avoiding violence, but about actively and constructively having the power to make a change for the better.

The hundreds of thousands of unnamed Indians working for independence were the impetus for the practice of nonviolence in action, known as *satyagraha*.

Satyagraha means "truth-force" or "love-force" that is the power behind nonviolent resistance, a term coined and used by Gandhi and the resistance movement for a free India (Gandhi, 1929).

Gandhi applied teachings from the seminal yoga text the *Bhagavad Gita* to the campaign to free India from British colonial rule. When he went to jail for civil disobedience, the text he brought with him was the *Bhagavad Gita* and he signed his letters from the jail Yeravda Mandir, or Yeravda Temple.

Using applied yoga, specifically the teachings of *ahimsa* and *satya* (nonviolence and truth), Gandhi created *satya-graha* or truth-force. *Satyagraha* encouraged people to find the power within themselves through yogic practices of self-discipline (*tapas*), focus (*dhyana*) and others, in order to help fight and overcome external rule.

REFLECTION

This method of nonviolent protest ignited the imagination and power of the Indian people and ultimately helped drive the British out of India. Critical to this method was the belief in *swaraj*, or self-rule. This is a clever play on words because Gandhi used *swaraj* with a double meaning. The first meaning is for Indians to use spiritual and yogic teachings to create sovereignty through living simply. The second meaning is self-rule as in political independence. Once a person was living more powerfully on a personal level it was easier to inspire thousands of people to take up campaigns for political autonomy. This gave rise to campaigns such as when Indians refused to buy the expensive British cotton and instead created homespun *Khadi* cloth. Or the salt march when thousands of Indians marched to protest the British tax on salt, an abundant natural resource, to highlight the absurdity of British rule and the inevitability of the coming Indian Independence.

Today, there are nonviolent practitioners all over the subcontinent who work in this legacy, preserving seeds to create biodiversity despite mono-cropping, teachers who are devoted to teaching students regardless of their class status, and those who seek to preserve a religiously diverse and democratic India despite its current movement toward religious fundamentalism and persecution of religious minorities. The need is still great, and many Indians in India still practice yoga in action as *swaraj* and *satyagraha* in their efforts to create social and political change.

Utilizing power with others is a method of building *sangha*, or spiritual community. Building *sangha* is an integral part of yoga practice.

Grappling with the questions in this text and knowing your position and commitments in the world and in yoga practice spaces are ways of cultivating power within.

REFLECTION QUESTIONS

- Where do you use the different types of power—power over, power with and power within?

- Where, specifically, do you see yoga and yogis being nonviolent?

- Where can you be nonviolent and practice *satyagraha*—truth-force?

YOGIS AND PRIVILEGE

As we examine power and reflect on our own role in overcoming separation, to get closer to yoga as unity, we must reflect on privilege.

It's the nature of privilege to not see that we have it. This is how systems of power and oppression perpetuate themselves. Privilege is the opposite side of oppression.

Privilege is defined as a special right or advantage or immunity granted or available only to a particular person or group (Tatum, 2007).

For example, an able-bodied thin person walking into a yoga studio may not consider that the steps she has to climb to reach the studio are a barrier for access to others. This is a way that her privilege is invisible to her. This same person may notice that in class, everyone looks more or less like her—thin, white, able-bodied and cisgender. These are privileges that enable her to feel at home, welcome and at ease in the yoga space.

However, if a queer, trans, disabled, bigger-bodied person of color tries to walk into that same space, they may immediately feel unwelcome by virtue of their lack of privilege, or target identities. They may not even be able to enter the space due to accessibility issues. Once in the space, they may not feel welcome or at ease, or may have more barriers to feeling that they belong.

Having privilege or not greatly shapes our day-to-day experiences. It has a vast influence on our lives. Privilege can either:

1. Be gained over time (i.e., having a college degree or getting a promotion)

   or

2. Be a societal construct based on things beyond our control (i.e., being born in a dominant country and free society, or being born white, or being born into wealth).

When we explore it in a yoga context, privileges from white privilege to cisgender or heterosexual privilege, to thin privilege to class privilege, all the ways we have or do not have privilege impact us moment-by-moment.

Explorations such as this are part of our practice of *svadhyaya*. *Svadhyaya* is the practice of self-inquiry and getting curious, having an open mind, engaging in critical thinking and exploring our own blind spots.

By beginning to look clearly at the ways we have or lack privilege, we pave the way for more caring action and more yoga as unity.

One important point is that many emotions may arise as we explore where we have or do not have privilege. It is common to feel guilty, but important not to get stuck in feeling guilty about all the ways we may have privilege. The power of realizing our privilege is leveraging it to help others who don't have the same access that we do. We help no one when we try to deny or avoid the privileges we have.

Facing the ways we have been targeted or oppressed can also be triggering and painful. Take great care with yourself as you engage in this reflection. Revisit the supportive steps for self or community care if they are helpful for you. Keep in mind that this is powerful and transformative work.

R
E
F
L
E
C
T
I
O
N

103

REFLECTION QUESTIONS

R
E
F
L
E
C
T
I
O
N

- Create a **Privilege/Target T-Chart** and label one side dominant or privilege and the other side target or disprivilege. Target represents the areas where you do not have institutional privilege or power. (See the Resource section at the end of the book for an example of my own privilege/target T-Chart.)

- Reflect and list for yourself where you may hold privilege and where your identity is targeted.

- How do you feel about where you may hold privilege?

- How do you feel about places where you may hold target identities?

- What feelings or questions does this exercise bring up for you?

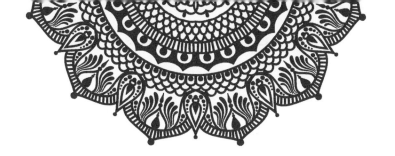

PART 2

BODY CULTURE, TOKENIZING AND WHITE CENTERING

"Art is the truth delivered through the medium of beauty."

— Mahadevi Verma

YOGIS AND WHITE CENTERING

As we explore privilege more deeply, we see that, in a system of white supremacy, the whole system is set up to center some and not others. This is what we call white centering. White centering is the idea that whiteness is normal, typical, right and expected.

For example, we see white centering when studio owners mostly or exclusively hire white teachers, spotlight them as experts and use white students in their marketing materials.

White centering happens when groups claim to be creating the first "yoga renaissance" when actually that renaissance happened time and again during South Asian history.

White centering also happens when a person of color brings up a cultural issue and a group of white people makes it about them. For example, I've heard white people respond to Indians raising concerns about appropriation by saying, "I studied in India, and my Indian friend says…" or, "I love India! There's no way I could be appropriating," or, "I have over 5,000 hours of training."

White centering is when a white teacher becomes the foremost hired and paid expert in Sanskrit even when there are countless South Asian Sanskrit scholars.

When you center whiteness in a tradition that has been practiced indigenously by Brown people, it erases the many Indians and other Brown and Black folks who taught and practiced yoga for centuries, as well as the Indians who shared yoga across the globe.

The information shared not only centers whiteness, but evokes a white savior narrative that is simply false and misleading, at best, racist and problematic, at worst. White saviorism is when white people believe the false narrative that they must save the poor, uncivilized brown savages. It serves to continue the idea of white as superior and Brown or Black as inferior, but cloak that idea in a story that makes white people feel great about the good they are doing for others.

White centering also revolves around the idea of white superiority, that whiteness and white people are better than others. Though this isn't an idea that most people will admit to, it is part of the "air we breathe," as Beverly Tatum (2007) says, and we need to explore this in order to address the causes of separation that stop us from achieving equity and unity.

When we look directly at all the ways yoga culture in the West centers whiteness, we begin to see more of what we might change.

INTERNALIZED OPPRESSION

Just as power can be internal, so can oppression. Internalized oppression is part of the insidious nature of power and it occurs when we internalize harmful and negative descriptions of ourselves as a target group. For many, internalized oppression is a kind of decentering of ourselves.

Internalized oppression is powerful. It affects our minds.

If a person of color internalizes the oppression of racism, they can begin to internalize that "not belonging" is actually their fault. They may feel inferior or less-than (the natural corollary to white centering and white supremacy).

In the recent Honor (Don't Appropriate) Yoga Summit, 100% of the South Asians I spoke with in the U.S. felt not at home or uncomfortable in yoga spaces. Most of the interviewees with marginalized identities have their own stories of exclusion within yoga spaces and communities (Barkataki, 2019).

Internalized oppression can look like critique of ourselves, our own people or other people of color. For example, colorism within the POC community, anti-immigrant sentiments by other immigrants, anti-blackness, self-assimilation, homophobia within the LGBTQ+ community, transphobia, etc.

POSSIBLE ACTIONS TO ADDRESS WHITE CENTERING

Whether we are in target identities or dominant ones, we can all address white centering. This work helps to undo internalized and external oppression.

R
E
F
L
E
C
T
I
O
N

For example, if all or the majority of the yogis you know, learn from and follow are white, diversify that. There are many South Asian / Indian and BIPOC people past and present from whom to learn.

We can center multiple South Asian teachers on our knowledge bases and platforms to combat their intentional and pervasive erasure in a yoga space. Diversity doesn't mean tokenization—it's not checking off a box, but rather a commitment to meaningful and substantial change in representation. When we pursue diversity in a tokenizing way, even without realizing it, it perpetuates the centering of white people and lumps all people of color into the Brown/Black category.

To truly diversify, you must look through a more human lens rather than a racial one. Diversity is about collaboration, differing opinions and co-creation. If you're surrounding yourself with only people who look like you or tokenizing the POC in the space to make yourself look better, you're missing the point.

REFLECTION QUESTIONS

* Where do you see white centering in the yoga community in the West? Let's get specific. If you work at a yoga studio or buy from yoga clothing companies, are all or the majority of the models white? Or do you generally practice with or alongside or hire white yoga teachers? At festivals or conferences are you attending the white teachers' workshops?

* Do you hold any feelings that whiteness or white teachers are superior to teachers of color?

* What can you do to help shift this in yourself or others?

YOGIS AND TOKENIZING

As we work to make our yoga spaces more equitable, we need to make sure we are not tokenizing in the process.

Tokenizing is treating a member of a group like they are a representative of the whole group (hooks, 2018). In yoga contexts, tokenizing is often steeped in the power structures of orientalism and colonialism. Orientalism—the treating of Asians and South Asians as the exotic "other"—is a stereotype that is often purported to be a "good thing." The reality is that stereotypes are never good.

Tokenization is common. When referring to Indians, it can sound like:

"Some of my best friends are Indian."

"Great people. So easy to corrupt, though."

"I asked my Indian friend and they said it is okay."

"So smart, so cooperative. So spiritual. Most eager-to-please I've ever met."

"All the Indians I know work so hard."

Racism isn't always as blatant as white nationalist rallies. Racism can be subtle, taking such forms as microaggressions, misnaming and tokenizing communities. This perpetuates an imbalance of power that has been present for generations.

Tokenizing is often used to look like we are creating more diversity. For example, tokenization can happen when a white-owned, run and dominated yoga space brings in one person of color but expects that person to simply conform to the culture that is already in place within the studio. In online spaces, in tele-summits or live events, the lineup will be all white teachers with one Brown teacher and perhaps one Black teacher. This is tokenization and it must be addressed and changed.

POSSIBLE ACTIONS TO ADDRESS TOKENIZATION

The first and most obvious way to address tokenization is to bring in a group or collective of people rather than just one person.

When this is done, time and care must be taken to ensure the institution is ready for the culture shifts that may occur when new norms are established.

Addressing and speaking up to point out tokenization works well when it is done kindly and firmly. I often find myself gently reminding people to be sure they are building relationships and including multiple points of view.

Another concrete way to address tokenization is to build relationships with the underrepresented and underestimated people you are working to include. When the relationships are strong, you can ask those folks what they think should be done.

Another concrete way to avoid tokenization is to build connection and community with more than one person of a particular demographic. For example, when I speak on panels I often request that the organizer hire other folks of color, other South Asians and do more to amplify representation rather than tokenize us.

REFLECTION QUESTIONS

- Where do you see tokenizing in yoga in the West?

- How might we respond in ways that don't tokenize?

- Brainstorm ways you can address tokenizing when you see it happening and what you might do instead.

YOGIS AND THE CULT OF BODY CULTURE

This misunderstanding and tokenization happen not only to people, but to yoga itself. Yoga is not simply the physical practice. *Asana*, or postures in yoga, seem to make up the majority of how yoga is typically represented in most studios, yoga spaces and online in the West.

You may think this is harmless. But actually, this reduction of yoga to focus on the cult of body culture has its roots in Western Enlightenment thinking. This equation of yoga with the body is a direct result of the split between mind and body that began in the 1600s, as described by philosopher Rene Descartes, when he said, "*Cogito, ergo sum*"—"I think, therefore I am" (Descartes, 2010).

In so saying, Descartes managed to describe the way Western civilization largely separated people from themselves and one another. This ideal gave rise to the Industrial Revolution and a direct focus on the body as separate from the psyche or soul.

It is this separation that we have carried over into yoga as we engage with it in the West.

Yoga is so much more than the poses.

If you aren't practicing ethics, integrating philosophy, practicing *seva*, kindness, self-reflection and meditation, working to uplift others, then it's important to ask: are you actually practicing yoga at all? *Asana* alone isn't all of what it means to practice yoga.

My teacher Shankara in the Shankaracharya tradition in Bihar used to say, "I really don't care just how perfect your pose is. I want it to feel well in your body, mind, spirit and soul!"

Yoga isn't simply something you do. It's something you are and that you can embody.

As we reflect on who is denied access to yoga, we can include reflection upon the banished, shamed or exiled parts of ourselves.

The harm caused by reducing yoga to just poses is hopefully clearer now.

By erasing history, indigenous ways of knowing and reducing the full practice of yoga to *asana*, we perpetuate a diminishing of the practice.

This also reduces the potential for the practice to support liberation for ourselves and for future humans.

The yoga we practice can mirror and reflect the society we are in, or transform it.

We can't separate the harm done now from that done during the colonization of India.

While on my research journey through Shimla, I spoke to a villager who said his own uncle and auntie (or ancestors) were punished and jailed for practicing yoga and *Ayurveda* during British rule.

These indigenous ways of liberating ourselves were punished under colonial rule. Condemning or eliminating the healthcare and wellness systems of a people is a common tool of war/violence/colonization. Yoga was often sanctioned, however, when it was reduced to mostly physical practice that suited the dominating group, in this case, the British.

Yoga defined as just poses is all around us, which is no wonder given the extent of colonial impact. This isn't permission to name-call, but to observe and reflect within and around you. To courageously and vulnerably share. Only when we really see what's happening can we begin to raise awareness to change it.

We will explore in Section Four how to avoid tokenizing yoga by learning the fullest extent of its expansive practice.

R
E
F
L
E
C
T
I
O
N

REFLECTION QUESTIONS

 Share stories and examples of where yoga is reduced to just poses. What need do you think this may fulfill for the person or institution reducing yoga in this way?

 This calls for brave reflection: Where have you seen yoga reduced to just poses and what do you or can you do instead?

 What is the cost of focusing exclusively on *asana* and what are the mind, body and spirit benefits of focusing on more of the eight limbs or other yogic practices?

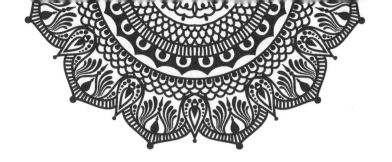

PART 3

ALLYSHIP AND ACCOMPLICESHIP

*"If you have come here to help me you are wasting your time,
but if you have come because your liberation is bound up with
mine, then let us work together."*

— LILLA WATSON

YOGIS AND ALLYSHIP

As we reflect on power and privilege, there are some helpful tools and roles that can support our practice of yoga as unity.

As Rafael Diaz argues in his essay "In These Times" (2017), "White supremacy has ensured that people of color have suffered the worst oppressions our country has to offer—from the genocide of Native Americans to slavery, Jim Crow, mass incarceration, deportation and the vast racial wealth gap… But White Americans continue to face high rates of suicide, poverty, debt, opioid overdoses and alcoholism. While these rates don't match the disproportionately high levels of suffering among people of color, our shared vision needs to be more than the racially equitable distribution of suffering: *All* suffering and injustice must come to an end."

Allyship can be the beginning of a helpful framework for doing the work of moving from separation toward unity. Here we will explore what it means to be an ally, co-conspirator or accomplice.

An aggressor or an oppressor is the originator of the oppressive situation or action. A bystander is someone who stands by and does nothing in the face of inequity or injustice. In contrast, an ally works alongside and supports someone who is targeted or experiences disprivilege. An ally works to support another.

To be an ally is to willingly step into leveraging one's privilege to address where others are marginalized. "An Ally is like a disrupter and educator in spaces dominated by Whiteness" (Whiteaccomplices.org, 2019). A co-conspirator listens to, builds community and works directly with the most impacted communities. An accomplice takes this work even further.

I first heard the language of allyship and accompliceship in the intentional activist community I built in Los Angeles from 2001 to 2015. We were an integrated group of people with intersectional identities working on dismantling racism, patriarchy, heteronormativity, classism and other forms of separation. We put the work of being an ally into practice as people who advocated for and supported members of a community other than our own by reaching across differences to uplift one another.

However, we soon found that allyship was not always enough. We began developing tools and praxis for how to be accomplices.

We realized that both allies and accomplices are necessary. Allies are committed to self-education and the education of others, while accomplices jump in and act alongside those who are targeted.

For example, an ally may educate herself about the prison-industrial complex and the school-to-prison pipeline.

An accomplice organizes and fundraises to stop incarceration rates among young people of color. An accomplice also may write letters or support getting those unjustly incarcerated out of the criminal justice system.

As we developed our work in this way, we learned from resources such as the 2014 essay on Indigenous Action Network (2014) that called for allies to move beyond mere allyship and join in the struggle alongside targeted people as accomplices.

We worked hard to call each other in, to call each other out, to do our work across lines of connection and division. We worked to show up for someone else's struggle, even if our own lives weren't impacted directly. To react and respond as an accomplice meant being there for our comrade as if their struggles were our own.

This concept of accompliceship vs allyship has continued to be developed in the wider sphere of those working to end oppression, such as in the work of Doran and Lebron (2019). One of the major differences between being an ally and being an accomplice is the extent to which someone addresses the systemic nature of the imbalance in power and oppression they are trying to change.

According to Teaching Tolerance (2017), "An ally will mostly engage in activism by standing with an individual or group in a marginalized community. An accomplice will focus more on dismantling the structures that oppress that individual or group—and such work will be directed by the stakeholders in the marginalized group."

For example, an ally may take it upon themselves to self-educate on a particular topic, say, the racist practice of redlining, a discriminatory practice that prevents poor/BIPOC from obtaining loans for houses in particular areas. An accomplice would instead go with a family who is being impacted by these racist practices to the bank and advocate on their behalf, or even co-sign on the loan.

In the yoga context, an ally may educate themselves on the issues of colonization and appropriation and bring up these topics in her studio or YTT group. An accomplice would also educate herself, then actively seek out organizations led by Desis or other Indian people, to pay, provide platforms for, listen to and learn from.

YOGIS AND PERFORMATIVE ALLYSHIP

Performative allyship is when someone acts as if they are trying to do the work of social and racial justice, but they are really acting in this way to avoid looking bad, or to self-promote and look good.

"The performatively woke person is someone whose desire to be seen as on the right side of an issue can get in the way of an ally's true job" (Peterson, 2017).

Often, performative allyship distracts from the issue at hand, takes the focus off the target or marginalized voices and in the worst cases can be harmful to the cause.

In "Guidelines for Being Strong White Allies," Paul Kivel directs us to, "notice who is at the center of attention and who is at the center of power" (Kivel, 2006).

As colleague Zahra Ali shared in a trauma-informed yoga teacher training at Ignite Yoga and Wellness Institute (2019), the target person or issue should be at the center of care. All those around that person or event should be lending support within. Support should radiate toward that issue or person.

That person at the center of the event should be able to ask for support and care from anyone involved—colleagues, allies, friends and so on—in the concentric circles around them. Those who are not at the impact point of the event should not ask for care, but instead offer support.

Performative allyship flips this and creates more stress on the person or issue at the center and diverts attention away from the issue.

There is a strong need and role for allies who are actively and thoughtfully engaging this work.

Deep reflection and continually coming back to your intentions will help you avoid acting as an ally in a performative way.

YOGIS AND VIRTUE SIGNALING

An important concept connected to performative allyship is virtue signaling. This is where yogis use things such as *namaste*, the *chakras*, or some other sign or symbol to imply their position as a spiritual teacher. These words and symbols, which are borrowed from another culture, are used to intentionally telegraph "enlightened wokeness."

Using a word such as "Bohemian" or "Indy" to reference Indians or "tribe" when you aren't actually Indigenous or First Nations doesn't signal your virtue. It signals your willingness to use another culture to prop up a certain image of yourself.

Ultimately, this is not the most inclusive, thoughtful way to communicate the message you may be after.

REFLECTION QUESTIONS

- Being direct and honest with yourself: Where in your life and practice are you more of a bystander, where are you more of an ally, and where are you more of an accomplice?

- Where have you seen performative allyship and virtue signaling?

- How can you self-assess to ensure you are moving toward care and support, rather than centering yourself, as you work for change?

YOGIS AND ACCOMPLICESHIP

You can further your Embrace Yoga practice by moving from allyship to co-conspiratorship to accompliceship. A co-conspirator works with and listens to a person or a group they are working to uplift.

An accomplice not only learns and educates about issues of inequity and structural injustice (as does an ally), an accomplice also gets involved, working to change the systems that causes harm.

As Colleen Clemens (2013) said, "An ally will mostly engage in activism by standing with an individual or group in a marginalized community. An accomplice will focus more on dismantling the structures that oppress that individual or group—and such work will be directed by the stakeholders in the marginalized group."

In May 2014, Indigenous Action Media published the anonymous essay, "Accomplices Not Allies: Abolishing the Ally Industrial Complex." This piece was intended to shake up the structure of how allyship work had been done and it offered a new framework for those with privilege to question their actions and act as accomplices.

For example, an ally may learn and teach themselves about the Indian roots of yoga, whereas an accomplice would also invite a South Asian or Indian teacher to share their knowledge. This accomplice may share the stage, platform and even a paycheck with the South Asian steward of yogic knowledge.

An ally would support Black Lives Matter and an accomplice would run classes as fundraisers for the cause and seek to defund the police or follow other calls from Black leadership. In so doing, the accomplice works to change the structures of how decisions are made and power is held.

REFLECTION QUESTIONS

◉ Give three examples of allyship and three examples of turning that into accompliceship.

◉ What might someone be nervous about when considering being an accomplice and how could you assuage those fears?

◉ What do you commit to as an ally and an accomplice in doing this work alongside BIPOC and South Asian stewards of yoga?

YOGIS AND SPIRITUAL BYPASSING

As we are reading, learning and working to change yoga culture in the West, we may encounter spiritual bypassing, so it is helpful to know what it is and how to address it. Spiritual bypassing is using spiritual concepts of unity to avoid or skip over current imbalances of power injustices rather than address them.

The term was coined by clinical psychologist John Welwood in 1983. He describes spiritual bypassing as using "spiritual ideas and practices to sidestep personal, emotional 'unfinished business' to shore up a shaky sense of self, or to belittle basic needs, feelings, and developmental tasks" (Welwood, 1983).

For example, if, in response to a person of color bringing up racial bias in a yoga studio, someone says, "Well, I don't see color," "We are all just one," or "All light and love," it sidesteps the serious and systemic issue that the person of color is raising. In a world where Black and Brown people are harmed every day just for their color, spiritual bypassing perpetuates this harm by refusing to acknowledge the very real and painful impacts of systems of oppression.

It can be easy and convenient to stay in a bypass position and say, "We are a welcoming studio and space. Everyone is welcome here." Yet when there are no Brown, differently-abled, bigger-bodied or trans people in leadership or other significant roles at your studio, retreat or class, the validity of such a statement must be examined.

Now one proviso is to consider where your studio or community may be highly homogenous, then it may be quite challenging to have more diversity in the studio space. However, there are a few considerations here. First, many places have more diversity than may be seen. It is important to seek out and connect with those who may be sidelined or living or working on the fringes. Secondly, much of the time, there are many facets of diversity that we can explore—body diversity, neurotypical diversity, diversity of ability and so on. Building authentic relationships is a cornerstone of developing this type of diversity so it is not tokenizing.

REFLECTION

Yoga is unity. But it is not simply unity in a pat or simplistic way. It is not a unity that denies difference. It is a unity that embraces and celebrates it, one that addresses separation and discrimination.

To practice and live in this world of unity, we must center ourselves in truth. This includes looking at the hard, challenging and unfair things about our world.

Many times spiritual bypassing happens because we are uncomfortable with holding space for someone else's truth. I like to ask in those moments, "What would it mean for you and your life if this were true?"

REFLECTION QUESTIONS

- What might you say to someone who uses spiritual terms such as, "We are all one," to bypass inequity?

- Where do you or others in your yoga practice or community practice performative allyship, virtue signaling or spiritual bypassing? Get specific about where you or others may perhaps have tried to spiritually bypass an uncomfortable truth.

- What supports you in holding space for someone else's truth even when it might be uncomfortable?

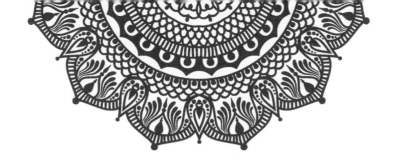

PART 4

EQUITY AND DIVERSITY

"To have self-mastery is to be a yogi."

—Mrigendra Tantra, 450 C.E. (E. Gangotri, 1999)

YOGIS AND AUTHENTIC LEADERSHIP

Leadership in yoga revolves around autonomy.

As stated in the *Mrigendra Tantra,* yoga invites a level of sovereignty over ourselves that means we embody what we learn, practice and teach.

We can remind ourselves that yoga isn't simply something you do, but is something you are. Instead of following the norms in the West where yoga is reduced to fitness, to images on social media, to a completely "outer" practice, we can go far beyond the poses and, in this way, embody our leadership.

As the texts teach us, yoga is an inner practice. It is a way of being. A way of living and engaging with life.

During the struggle for Indian Independence, many who practiced civil disobedience were guided to explore *swaraj*, or self-rule. As we've discussed, this practice of *swaraj* has a double meaning. It is a practice of finding autonomy and self-mastery within through spiritual practice. It is also the practice of autonomy as a populace capable of governing itself. The key to Indian Independence from the colonizing British is that when enough of a population has inner self-rule, there is no way an outer force can hold it down. This was one of the basic tenets of the struggle for independence, and it applies to us today.

True leadership comes from within. Yoga is the means to this inner leadership.

In many of the yogic texts, such as the *Bhagavad Gita*, as practitioners of yoga we are invited to have control over ourselves and our senses. We are also asked to give our actions up and not be attached to their fruits, such as in the *Bhagavad Gita* chapter 2, verse 48.

"Perform every action abandoning attachment. Give every action up. Be equal in success or failure. This equanimity is yoga."

Practicing yoga in this way can be an act of leadership.

If every action you take is done with devotion, everything from the mundane, the ordinary and the dirty chores to washing and adorning the altars can become an act of care.

When every action is love embodied, of serving something greater than yourself, of moving toward equity, then you are always practicing yoga.

This is the leadership of yoga in action.

REFLECTION QUESTIONS

What kind of leaders have you seen in yoga in the West and what beneficial qualities does a yoga leader embody?

Where are you moving into yoga leadership, both on inner and outer levels?

What gaps might you have in your leadership growth?

REFLECTION

YOGIS AND COLONIZATION
AND DECOLONIZATION

*"Holding the great bow of yogic wisdom, the aspirant
should fix the arrow of mind, sharpened with meditation,
on its target. Draw the string with full absorption and
shoot at the target. My friend, remember immutable,
eternal Truth alone is the target."*

MUNDAKA UPANISHAD 2.2.3

COLONIZATION

To engage a process of decolonization, we must address the causes of colonization.

The Oxford English Dictionary (2018) defines colonization as, "the action or process of settling among and establishing control over the indigenous people of an area. As well as the action of appropriating a place or domain for one's own use."

Colonization has occurred in many different circumstances and its impacts are far-reaching.

Kēhaulani (2016) argues that colonization is not just a one-time event or something that happens over time, but a system that exists and influences cultural and social institutions.

In Colonial India, the British not only established control, but extended that control in various ways.

According to the book *The Sword of Tippu Sultan* by K.L. Kamat, "From 1616 when the British East India Company entered Bombay, and under 'Crown Rule' from 1858 until 1947, colonizing powers, such as the British, took the land of colonies, utilized and exploited the labor, natural resources, industrial power, and anything else they could find of value in India to their own benefit without regard to the native population causing oppression."

In a system and context where colonial oppression has taken away agency to practice indigenous and native healing and strengthening practices such as yoga, we must remember that colonization of yoga is not just a metaphor. It's a practice that perpetuates a relationship of exploitation, taking power away from some while those in a position of power benefit from the stealing of natural resources and labor, as well as the ideas and cultural knowledge of indigenous people.

Some believe yoga exists in a post-colonial context. While others, including myself, believe yoga is practiced in a neo-colonial context. Post-colonial means that colonization has ended. Neo-colonial means that colonization has not ended, but it has continued and changed forms.

For those of us who are Indian or from colonized people and places, our families and spiritual lineages may have been fractured and wisdom hidden or lost.

For those of us who have ancestors who were colonizers, we may have been cut off from our own cultures, as well as from our sense of connection, compassion and humanity.

Colonization causes harm to all because any time there is oppression, it harms both the oppressed and the oppressor.

The devastating separating power of oppression is that it prevents connection. It divides us from our ability to connect with others.

It also divides us from the ability to connect with ourselves.

We are sharing and practicing a yogic tradition that has been impacted by colonization, and we ourselves have likely also been impacted by colonization in some form.

This context of neo-colonial harm is one that needs attention and care and gives rise to the need for the work of decolonization in yoga.

DECOLONIZING YOGA

Just like colonization, decolonization is a process as well as an outcome. It is multilayered, and it happens over time.

Decolonization is first and foremost the return of land to the indigenous people from whom it's been stolen (Tuck and Yang, 2016).

Tuck and Yang write of the United States context of settler colonialism where the colonists arrived, took over land from indigenous people and will never leave. Their claim is that for decolonization to happen, land must be returned to indigenous stewardship.

In our practice with yoga, decolonization is also not just a metaphor. Decolonizing can take the form of acting in restoration of that sovereignty, resources, goods, wealth, land, spiritual riches, power and knowledge.

Decolonization is connected to working to re-indigenize or create reparations on multiple levels for those most impacted. It can be complex and multilayered.

In yoga, to indigenize means not only to return the power and control to those from whom the cultural knowledge and practices came, but also to elevate and embrace the cultural elements indigenous to original yoga practice.

Some keys for decolonization are to:

- Include indigenous perspectives, values and cultural respect in daily practices. For example, ask Indian practitioners to share their experiences with yoga. Travel to a context where South Asian people are gathered and join them in their territory, in their experience of practicing yoga or merging with the divine.

- Another example of decolonizing our yoga practice can come through something concrete like the music that we play if we play music in yoga *asana* class. Traditionally, yoga *asana* was practiced in silence. However, in some contexts, music is used. In many yoga classes in the West, we have music that is not connected to the tradition at all being played. Or, also we may see traditional music, such as *bhajans* or *kirtan*, being performed by white Western practitioners, who may not have the pronunciation or context correct for the cultural context. So, we can learn more about the context; Indian, Desi, South Asian musicians and artists; and if we are going to play music, we can include music from practitioners from within the tradition.

- Thoughtfully position indigenous knowledge, which comes from the land and the people and their stories and ways of knowing at the heart of all that we do.

- Include cultural practices in the operations of our schools, studios and institutions.

To be colonized is to become a stranger in your own land. This is the feeling many Indian people have in most Westernized yoga spaces today.

This colonization of yoga happens when the full, complex breadth of yoga's intention for the practice of liberation is reduced to less than its many limbs.

Yoga is not a practice intended to perfect physical strength or skill as its main aim. It is not a practice aimed at reducing stress so we can be cogs in a wheel of production and consumption.

Yoga's many aims involve developing the skills of transcendence. The practices, such as the limb of *asana*, aim at strengthening the body in order to practice absorptive states of meditation.

The aim of this kind of meditative awareness is to experience, practice and live oneness of mind, body and soul with the divine. This kind of freedom is called *samadhi,* or liberation. It is painful that a practice meant to free us has becoming so limiting.

Decolonization is a far-reaching process. It is iterative and changes and evolves over time.

We must work toward repairing the harm caused in order to practice decolonization.

R
E
F
L
E
C
T
I
O
N

REFLECTION QUESTIONS

🌸 How are we harmed by colonization even today?

🌸 What is decolonization?

🌸 Why is decolonization not just a metaphor? What are concrete ways we can begin or continue to decolonize our practice?

YOGA AND DIVERSITY, INCLUSION, ACCESSIBILITY AND THE MOVEMENT TOWARDS EQUITY

As we move from reflecting on the causes of separation toward creating unity, we must create some understanding and tools to bring equity into yoga. We have many opportunities to create equity in person, on-line, in collaboration and mutual uplift.

We will break down common terms, such as inclusion, diversity and accessibility so we can begin to put these concepts into useful action.

A reminder for context: As we discussed above in the section on "Separation," yoga in the West is not diverse. Yoga has a "look," and that look is not representative of diversity. Diversity in practice is often used to essentially mean tokenization.

Diversity means respecting, including and celebrating differences. These can be along the dimensions of race, ethnicity, gender, sexual orientation, socio-economic status, age, physical abilities, religious beliefs, political beliefs or other identifying factors (Tatum, 2003).

WHAT DIVERSITY MISSES

Diversity takes a tally of who is there and who is not. However, it does not necessarily address the way an experience serves people with various structural, systemic or interpersonal needs.

To put this another way, diversity addresses numbers and access. It does not address the quality of the environment and how it serves or does not serve those most impacted by systemic oppression.

Diversity is important. But if we stop with only diversity, we miss the mark.

R
E
F
L
E
C
T
I
O
N

YOGA AND INCLUSION

Inclusion is an intention or policy of including people who might otherwise be excluded or marginalized, such as those who are disabled or non-neuro-typical, or racial and sexual minorities.

Inclusion, like diversity, is a step in a better direction, but often is problematic. Though well-intentioned, inclusion presumes there is a group that is in power that has the ability to "bring in" others with less power. This is often a white normative group, so this approach becomes white centering. It uplifts the white power-holders and power-brokers as the ones at the center of the narrative who get to pick and choose who they "include," while they get rewarded for being "inclusive."

An analogy for why inclusion is problematic is when we say, "Invite us to the table." Who owns the table? Who sets the rules, manner and way things happen at the table? Contrast this to a model where the disadvantaged people create, set and furnish their own table.

YOGA AND ACCESSIBILITY

Accessibility refers to the design of products, devices, services or environments for people who experience disabilities. Accessibility in yoga focuses on how to make yoga teachings available to all, regardless of ability (Heyman, 2019).

There are many norms and practices in yoga culture in the West that make yoga inaccessible. From the plethora of acrobatic yoga selfies on Instagram to the teachers who demo at the extreme ends of the practice or make their students feel less-than for not being able to practice a particular version of a pose, yoga *asana* has become a vehicle for showing off physical accomplishments.

Accessibility in yoga is an incredibly important practice. My early teachers in yoga *asana* always described there being no one perfect pose. The perfect pose was the one that the student could get into and breathe deeply, fully and find some peace.

YOGA AND EQUALITY

Equality is the idea that everyone is the same and should be treated the same.

In yoga context in the West, we see this often when teachers impose the same alignment cues on a class, even when the students present a multiplicity of differing experiences, body histories, shapes, sizes, trauma and injury backgrounds, life stories and experiences.

WHAT EQUALITY MISSES

Equality sounds good, but does not serve us all. What equality misses is the fact that we don't all start from the same place, nor are we all the same, so we don't all need the same things. Equality imposes an inaccurate flattening of our unique experiences and backgrounds, leaving some (or many) of us underserved.

YOGA AND EQUITY

Equity is giving everyone what they need to be successful, taking into account the vast diversity of structural privilege, power and oppression, and life experience. Equity identifies and strives to eliminate blocks that have prevented some groups or people from participating fully.

Equity addresses systems and root causes, not just individuals and isolated events (Kapila, Hines and Searby, 2016).

Now I will examine some particular ways that we can make yoga more inclusive, accessible, diverse and equitable.

YOGA INSTITUTIONS AND BUSINESSES

Equity in a yoga institution or business can include implementing need-based scholarships and payment plans.

Need-based scholarships adjust for interlocking, generational and systemic inequity that impacts people's class status. For example, offering

R E F L E C T I O N

135

a varying rate scale based on what people can pay (sliding scale or variable donation).

For a course or workshop, you can set up tiered pricing where the Sustainer rate is the true cost, and a Supporter pays an additional sum to help subsidize the Equity and Justice rate. You can invite people to pay at the rate that is appropriate for them.

Supporter—$200 (to support oneself and someone else)

Sustainer—$150

Equity and Justice—$100

Another way to offer need-based scholarships is to offer partial or full scholarships. I and other trainers have found that it is important for folks to make some investment, however small, into a training or course in order for them to be accountable to it.

Equity in yoga can also look like diversifying boards of institutions, studios, training programs and yoga-based institutions.

When diversifying a board or leadership, it is important not to tokenize, for example, by bringing on one queer person, trans person or one person of color. This can lead to more harm. Instead, it can be effective to bring in groups, teams and multiple folks of varying identities.

Collaboration over competition is key. The new way (and also yogic way) of creating mutual uplift is to understand that we all rise together and work to support one another. It is important to focus on building relationships as part of this equity process. Relationships are built over time, by practicing *satya*, truthfulness, and cultivating conversations.

RETREATS AND FESTIVAL MODELS

Yoga retreats and festivals are in dire need of re-imagining. For many festivals and retreats, the lineup is representative of a mono-culture. One way to diversify this is to invite a number of teachers of color.

For example, at one yoga retreat, the founder, a teacher of color, creates a space that centers teachers of color, but is welcoming to all. This event is one where presenters are paid and real conversations, as well as teachings, happen on a deep level. It is important that teachers from disadvantaged backgrounds get paid well as they are often asked to do much free labor, plus they face the interlocking systemic struggles of economic racism.

It is important to consider acknowledging the lineage of the spiritual path you are teaching as well as the people who are indigenous to the land where you may be hosting the retreat. Consider how you can make reparations and support locals, by giving them positions of power and paying them well. It is also important to hold space with *ahimsa* and allow for complexity to emerge and be integrated in the retreat process.

STUDIOS

Equity in yoga studios looks like a studio doing their best to create equal access to folks in their community. Equity is giving students and teachers what they need to succeed, depending on from where they are starting and the conditions they are experiencing.

Within a yoga studio, equity can look like including lots of props, bolsters, blankets, chairs and other tools to make the practice available. Equity in a studio can also look like giving non-normative teachers prime time teaching positions and spots.

In yoga studio leadership, yoga businesses and at teacher trainings, equity can look like more training in culturally competent yoga, trauma-informed yoga or yoga for people with physical disabilities, along with training on creating safer and braver spaces.

YOGA CLASSES

In a yoga class, either in person or on-line, equity can look like the flexibility to alter a class based on the needs of the students that day.

Within a class where there are various needs, teach to the practitioner with the greatest need.

R
E
F
L
E
C
T
I
O
N

For example, a colleague, Jacoby Ballard, describes equity in a yoga class looking like centering the student with the greatest need and providing opportunities for other students to build leadership from within the foundation of their own practice.

"I teach in a cancer center where there might be a new student who has just received a cancer diagnosis practicing alongside someone with a very established practice. I ask everyone what they need for their body, but no one is required to reveal their status. As far as creating equity, I center the newer student in the class. Sometimes they can get on the floor and sometimes they can't. They may need practice relearning balance. I just do the simplest version of the pose, boiling down the essence of the pose. I know the person with the established practice will go into the version of the pose that serves them, but that is not what I am teaching."

Another colleague, Hala Khouri, who has taught *asana* for over a decade, guides her studio class like this: "If you want the simplest version of the pose do this. If you'd like a more complicated version do this. Sometimes the greatest medicine is to actually slow down and do less. Some of us do need a kick to do more. Choosing how to be in a pose is part of the practice."

Equity is often communicated through ample use of verbal, emotional and physical supports. This might look like cueing in an invitational way, or offering options. It also looks like having two blocks, a blanket, a strap, chair or wall available to support my own or my students' practice.

Equity in yoga *asana* classes is often realized by spending time before and after class listening to the students and their needs and adjusting according to the needs expressed in the moment.

TEACHER TRAININGS

The training of teachers is a complex issue and a huge responsibility. We are imparting yogic knowledge for future generations. It is a complex matter because traditionally yoga was taught in the *Gurukul* model, in very small groups or one to one. The sharing of yoga has popularized and modernized,

R
E
F
L
E
C
T
I
O
N

as well as commercialized, today. It is a position of great responsibility and not to be abused or taken lightly.

As yoga teachers and trainers today, it is key to acknowledge that we are not *gurus*. Most of us are not following that same traditional structure of instruction. However, we still have a responsibility to the tradition. It is important to train students in the entire breadth of what yoga is, not simply *asana*. In doing this, it is important to ensure that the teachers of trainings do their best to embody what they are teaching.

It is important to have teachers teach who they are and what they know. For example, teacher trainings bring me in to teach about yoga philosophy, cultural appropriation and yoga history and bringing yoga alive today, as someone who is an Indian teacher sharing the wisdom of my ancestors.

And for the teacher trainings that I run, there is a segment on Trans Justice and Trans-Inclusive Teaching. Though I may feel somewhat educated on this topic, and aspire to be an ally and accomplice, I make every effort to ensure this segment of my YTT is taught by a trans yoga teacher.

For example, yoga educator Jacoby Ballard joins virtually to run a workshop and guide my classes. It is important to me to pay consultants well, especially when it is someone who is often targeted for their identity teaching about the topic.

There is a different type of emotional labor that is involved when someone is teaching in an area where their identity has perhaps been a past source of trauma or targeted part of their identity.

Bring in a teacher representative of the issue being taught, both to support folks doing this work and because of the direct experience they bring to the topics at hand.

Teacher trainings as a whole can be served by bringing in much more content on the whole expanse of what yoga is, as well as including diversity, equity and inclusivity. Addressing appropriation in trainings helps prepare teachers to include and welcome all in their classes, as well as teach in a way that embraces yoga's roots.

REFLECTION

MARKETING AND ADVERTISING

As you put together your marketing and advertising materials, it is important to consider inclusivity and equity. Marketing and advertising are a key and important part to creating equity within a yoga business setting.

Know that who you put on the flyer or image will be the people who show up. Consider carefully who you choose to visually represent your event, workshop or training.

Second, if you put people of color on your flyer, but are not providing platforms for teachers of diverse backgrounds, this is tokenizing and misleading. Please ensure your marketing reflects truly equal representation!

These are some basic initial considerations on our path of creating more inclusivity, diversity and equity. Equity in yoga is something we must work not to tokenize, but to continually grow in and to explore and create together.

REFLECTION

REFLECTION QUESTIONS

- Do you understand the difference between equity and equality?

- Have you focused more on diversity and inclusion than working toward equity?

- What might you do to facilitate true equity in your yoga spaces?

V
RECONNECTION

"Whatever lessens suffering in yourself and others, that is right. Whatever increases suffering, that is wrong. The answer is within you. When you are free of pride and prejudice, when you are calm and attentive, a light will shine within you. Through meditation and through being mindful you will find your own knowledge of rightness. You will be your own light."

—Satish Kumar, *The Buddha and the Terrorist*

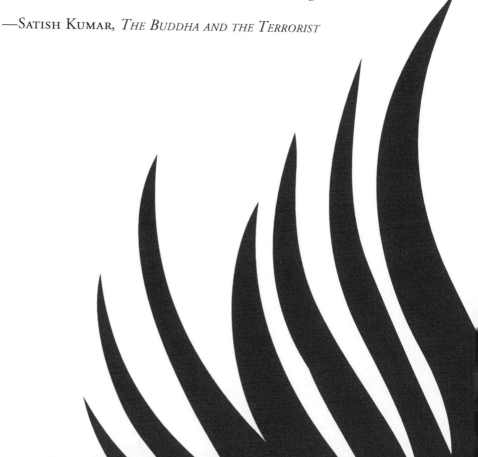

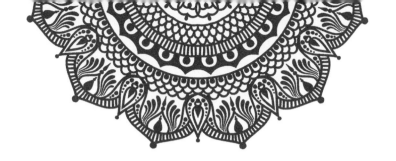

PART 1

RECONNECTION
IN ACTION

"All the suffering in the world comes from seeking pleasure for oneself. All the happiness in the world comes from seeking pleasure for others."

—SHANTIDEVA

THESE WORDS SPOKEN BY *SHANTIDEVA*, A BUDDHIST MONK AND SCHOLAR at *Nālandā* University in India around 700 C.E., resonate today.

We have come together through the path of reflecting deeply on the many blocks to unity and have begun to see the path toward unity and reconnection.

We've identified many of the causes of separation and seen how they come alive and operate in the world around us. We have reflected on where they show up in our lives. Now we can integrate what we have learned.

Based on yogic teachings, we will turn toward considering solutions for this problem of separation and creating true unity.

In this section we will explore some specific, concrete skills for doing the work of living and practicing yoga as unity that come from within the yogic tradition.

Not all tools will speak to everyone. But at least some of these tools will speak to you as practices you can begin to implement today, this week and into the future as you work to end separation, build your skills and capacity, and bring forth the world of yoga as unity.

YOGIS, CULTURAL APPRECIATION, POWER BALANCING AND AHIMSA

As an antidote to cultural appropriation, let's explore the skills of cultural appreciation, power balancing and *ahimsa* (non-harm).

We know that to create more equity we don't want to appropriate, so understanding what cultural appreciation is and how we can do it is key.

I often get asked the question, "If I am a white person should I teach yoga?" No one outside of yourself can answer that question for you. I will advocate for you to apply the practice of *viveka*, of wise discrimination and deep inquiry. Utilizing some of the tools in this book, as well as the support of cultural appreciation, may help guide your exploration.

Cultural appreciation seeks to connect with cultures different from one's own from the inside out.

It respects the codes, values and practices of the culture. Cultural appreciation can happen when one enjoys or respects the culture of origin. Instead of harming or taking, one learns with humility, gives back and uplifts the source culture.

Remember that to be present, cultural appropriation has two criteria:

1. Power imbalance
2. Causing harm

Similarly, cultural appreciation involves two criteria of power balancing and *ahimsa* (non-harm or harm reduction).

1. Power balancing: Sharing power or using privilege or advantage to uplift or support an under-resourced group or people. This is an appropriate use of *shakti*, or power.

2. Non-harm (*ahimsa*): Reducing or mitigating harm, or actively uplifting the source culture and its people. Consideration, care and respect that come from learning about and uplifting the source culture and those who often don't receive support. This can include financial, social, political, emotional and cultural care and support (Barkataki, 2015).

For example, examining one's privilege and using it to lift others up is a form of balancing power. I experienced this when I was a young organizer in my early 20s. I attended a meeting to help organize an anti-war march. Those in attendance were mostly white men in their 40s. My friend and I were the only people of color and we were both in our mid-20s. I was inexperienced in that space. My friend was a confident young man. I assumed he would step up and help lead the march we were organizing together and that I would help from behind the scenes.

As discussions unfolded on who would run the peace-keeping team for the march, I heard my friend say, "I think she should be our head peace-keeper," pointing at me.

In that moment, I was terrified. I didn't feel capable of leading much, let alone an entire peace march of what turned out to be more than 100,000 people. I tried to deflect. My friend insisted.

In the end, I did indeed lead the peace-keeping team on that historic march. And, though terrifying, it was a good thing I was leading, because someone with significant compassion and care was needed to break up a fight between pro-war and anti-war protestors. It turned out that my calm demeanor, fresh from the meditation cushion, helped calm a tense situation from becoming an out-and-out fight.

R
E
C
O
N
N
E
C
T
I
O
N

I never would have volunteered for that position, and none of the usual leaders would have chosen me. It was my friend, who chose to use his male privilege in that moment to speak up and give power over to the youngest, Brownest woman in the room, who changed the course of that march and of my life.

I learned not only that I could lead a march and keep the peace, but that sometimes having a voice that other people listen to means speaking up and using it not to claim power for oneself, but to pass the power to someone else.

This is a lesson I haven't forgotten and one that I carry with me as a reminder of sharing power.

NON-HARM: CONCRETE ACTIONS FOR CULTURAL APPRECIATION, NOT APPROPRIATION

Coming toward a tradition with openness, willingness to listen, respect and humility are wonderful ways to engage mutual exchange. We must avoid harm and address power imbalances.

- First and foremost, address your impact, not just your intention. Consider whether your actions may be causing harm and try to reduce that harm.
- Another powerful way to avoid appropriation is to embrace yoga's roots. Learn about the culture from the inside out. Explore the lineages. Explore the expanse of this practice far beyond just the physical. Read the *sutras* and cite sources of these wisdom teachings.
- If you are a yoga practitioner, ask your teachers for more than *asana*. Go deeper. Ask and take the time to learn and practice more.
- Practice and teach as many of the limbs and other aspects of yoga as possible so we can experience the full range of what yoga has to offer.
- We can own our positionality and honor our lineage. At the beginning of a yoga class, teachers can share, "This is who I am, this is how I learned; I have a lot of respect for the lineage…"

- Actively uplift. Centralize those who have been left out. Consider yoga's legacy and traditions, and what we may be missing by historical and present-day omission. We South Asians, Indians and Desis are here. Include us. Centralize us. Ask us. Invite us in. Lift us up. For example, if you are attending or hosting a yoga festival or conference, in-person or online, ensure that there are multiple South Asian wisdom holders speaking, teaching or otherwise represented in the lineup. Historical oppression and omission have taken from us a centralized position and a voice that should be ours to share. Include us and know there's room for you in the circle and in the practice.

- Be committed to studentship—practicing and teaching as we are always students of this practice. Act as if we could study it for our whole lives and always be learning, because, of course, we can. A little humility, a little reverence, goes a long way.

- Honor symbols and iconography. Make sure if we are using images of deities or regalia such as statues, *malas* (prayer beads) or *bindis* (spiritual adornment), that we know where they came from, what they mean, how to relate to them respectfully and have a sincere intention at heart. Deepening our relationship is key.

- Avoid exploitation. Show that we really care about others' wellbeing. This is not just a thing we are doing. Consider if you are profiting off another culture's wisdom and practices how you might make material reparations.

- Engage in courageous conversations at yoga sites. For example, you can connect with people at your studio or wherever you practice and engage in conversations around exploring yoga and cultural issues. These conversations aren't always comfortable, but they invite us to deal with the real. We must make space to lean into hard conversations such as these. We must reach for each other as we change ourselves and the world. We are all connected.

- We can explore questions such as:

- Where might we be appropriating yoga in our actions, practices, classes, merchandise? What might we do differently?
- What aspects of yoga culture and practice are we strong in practicing?
- What aspects can we deepen and practice more fully?
- What are some areas of growth and learning we can embrace as a community?

Appreciation involves awe, respect, reverence and humility. Just like you'd look at a raging river delivering sustenance to old growth forests and cities for centuries, knowing the river has been here before you, and knowing it's going to continue long and strong and beautiful after you are gone. This perspective invites awe and humility, not ownership and control. We can look at yoga with the same reverence.

Identify and reflect on your power, bring large amounts of compassion for yourself and others into this practice.

REFLECTION QUESTIONS

- What is the difference between cultural appropriation and cultural appreciation in your own words?

- What is one act of cultural appreciation you can do right now that will balance power or share power and provide care?

- How can you practice *ahimsa* (non-harm, non-violence) as you keep learning, exploring and visiting the wellspring of deep awe in this practice?

YOGIS AND HEALING JUSTICE

Yoga is a system of personal and social liberation and healing that should be available to all.

Healing justice is a practice that acknowledges our illnesses or maladies are not individual events, but are socially created, so healing must take into account justice in order to create wellness.

"Healing justice as a movement and a term was created by queer and trans people of color and in particular Black and Brown femmes, centering working-class, poor, disabled and Southern/rural healers" (Piepzna-Samarasinha, 2016).

The idea of healing justice is not new. Before we had a term for it, indigenous people—our grandparents and ancestors—were healing and supporting people in homes and civic spaces.

Part of the power of healing justice as a movement is reclaiming these roots and origins.

"If it's not centering Black / Indigenous / people of colour (BIPOC) healers, it's not healing justice. If it's not affordable, it's not healing justice" (Piepzna-Samarasinha, 2016).

Yoga is a healing tool and system that should be available to all, regardless of race, color, gender, sexual orientation, religion, ability or any other background.

But this is not the reality for many people.

Yoga culture in the West desperately needs a healing justice lens.

Black and Brown folks are disproportionately affected by heart disease, high blood pressure, diabetes, high maternal death rates, violence, suicide and other afflictions, according to the U.S. Department of Minority Health (2019). At the same time they are not represented in wellness or yoga.

We simply don't have representation or access to wellness tools that can help us get healthy, stay healthy or heal. If we don't see folks like us doing healthy things, it's hard to learn.

The U.S. Department of Minority Health (2019) notes Native and Black Americans have a death rate from heart disease that is 1.5 times higher than whites. South Asians are four times more likely to develop heart disease and almost one in three will die from heart disease before age 65. Black Americans are 77% more likely than white Americans to be diagnosed with diabetes. Latinxs have a 66% greater chance of developing heart disease, and one in three live with diabetes.

These inequities are furthered by the exclusion of yoga from certain communities.

We can begin to heal the harm caused by colonization and appropriation when we begin to address accessibility as a social justice issue. This is the inherent work of yoga as healing justice.

This means the practice of yoga must be opened up to everyone; anything else does not truly serve the aims of yoga.

REFLECTION QUESTIONS

⚙ What is healing justice and what is the relationship between yoga and healing justice?

⚙ Where can you support, uplift, collaborate with or provide platforms for other healers/teachers of color?

⚙ What organizations in your community (particularly organizations led by BIPOC) can you learn about, connect with and support?

R
E
C
O
N
N
E
C
T
I
O
N

YOGIS AND RADICAL CIVIC ENGAGEMENT PRACTICE

Yogic civic engagement invites a joyful paradox. Civic engagement invites us to get involved and to act *within* the world without getting too attached to being *of* the world.

Civic engagement is connecting, acting and caring beyond the sphere of our own lives, into a wider circle of influence and impact.

Yoga practitioners have, for thousands of years, responded, reacted to and sought freedom from constraint and oppression. For example, in early pre-Vedic times (around 100 BCE and earlier), when practitioners receded to the fringes of society and left the ease and joys of village and city life to find a deeper liberation than material comforts could offer them. Additionally, in response to various invasions by the Aryans, Mughals, and later the Christians, yoga and yogis persisted in a practice that would lead them to freedom and self-mastery.

Yoga, at its heart, is a radical and civically engaged practice.

Yoga is not now, nor has it ever been, a practice aimed at physical mastery for its own sake.

Shankara, my teacher in Bihar, India, taught that early yogis practiced on the fringes of society, both literally and figuratively. They were under trees, in caves, by rivers and streams.

They looked around at all the advancements organized city life had brought them some 2,500+ years ago (and Indian civilization was highly advanced, so it was quite a lot even then). But the yogis weren't content with mere sensory pleasures and delights and ease of the world, so they sought a kind of freedom beyond the confines of what society and its norms had to offer.

Today, we work with a reformulation: yoga = physical prowess + body worship. The physical practice was developed to break the attachment and connection to the physical body, not to deepen it. Now, we also utilize yoga and mindfulness to create passive worker-enhanced productivity in the illusory game of big business.

Further, students' "mindful" silence is called noble, but it is really mindfully manufactured compliance. Ronald Purser (2017) speaks of this when he says, "Mindfulness has been reduced to a privatized self-help technique that reinforces systems of oppression and injustice." We're simply contributing to the yoga-mindfulness-industrial complex.

Let's not forget that yoga and meditation practice has often been counter-culture. Both then and now.

Its aims were nothing short of total personal and social transformation.

Many yogis and *rishis* were concerned about the ills befalling early villages and cities as they started to urbanize. They developed practices and tools to share with the populace to keep the mind, body and spirit in harmony despite external conditions. These teachings are part of what we inherit as practitioners of the yogic path.

In the next section we will explore some tools for action. We now are in a time where our civic engagement is needed more than ever. We don't need to save the whole world, if that is not our calling. Our yogic tools give us a path toward engaging exactly where we are, with whom is in front of us.

R
E
C
O
N
N
E
C
T
I
O
N

REFLECTION QUESTIONS

Where do you see yoga and/or mindfulness being used to suppress rather than spur civic engagement?

What are you doing to get to the radical—as in the root(s)—of your practice?

How can you improve upon civic engagement in your community and how is yoga philosophy supportive of civic engagement?

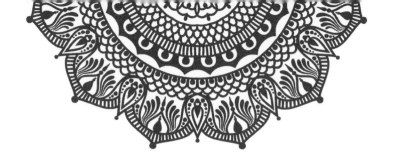

PART 2

RECONNECTION PRACTICES

"Uniformity is not nature's way; diversity is nature's way."

—Vandana Shiva

YOGIS AND PROVIDING PLATFORMS

Who we raise up and provide platforms for in our society and how we do that is important as we do this work.

As we addressed in the section on separation above, the power structure works in such a way that when you exclude those from whom the teachings came it makes it easier to erase, and then take positionality, steal and exploit this indigenous wisdom.

When you exclude people from whom this medicine came, it perpetuates exploitation and colonization in a global marketplace.

One way we can act to make yoga more inclusive and diverse is to address the issue of representation by providing access to those who don't typically get a platform.

There are many ways we can do this.

Start by considering who is normally not given a platform in yoga spaces. Begin to invite them in, uplift them, celebrate them. There are many ways to do this.

FOR YOGA STUDENTS

If you are a yoga student, you can frequent classes by people who normally don't get the primetime spots or who may not fit the yoga "norm." You can ask the studio manager to give that teacher or those teachers more classes or more primetime spots. You can subscribe to podcasts, take online classes and consume media by teachers with diverse experiences and backgrounds.

Speak up at events and gatherings where there isn't equal representation. In the resources section of this book I have included a general letter that you can send to events, festivals or yoga retreats that you can modify and email or send to organizers to request greater representation.

FOR YOGA TEACHERS

If you are a teacher, you can ask your studio to hire and promote your non-normative colleagues.

As a yoga teacher, part of your role is to practice and embody yoga ethics, so speaking up and addressing issues of disparity, appropriation and harm, when and if you feel able to do so, is crucial to your position.

FOR YOGA STUDIOS AND SCHOOLS

If you are a studio owner or yoga school, it is critical that you address these issues. Hire faculty who are teachers of diverse color, size, ability, sexuality and gender.

Develop a board of directors who can help bridge relationships between your studio and different community partners. There are many organizations and not-for-profits working in many regions that are already doing great work. Connect with them. Have a diversity of people on your board.

The truth is, for many of us, who we know impacts what we are able to achieve and experience. We can assess our own power and privilege, as well as our own target identities, and act accordingly.

As a personal example, so many of the opportunities I've gotten have been because a white ally got invited to a space, then lifted me up. In turn, I try to do this for others. For example, when I am invited in as a cis woman and I don't see trans perspectives addressed by trans people in a space, I advocate for the organization hiring a trans educator.

There is nothing to be lost by suggesting, providing platforms for and bringing in colleagues.

Gratitude and success are sweeter when shared.

Dare to lift up a yogi who is not normally in the spotlight. Shine a big light. Hire them. Suggest them as a speaker or teacher. Appreciate them!

Together, let's hold the vision of all yoga festivals, conferences, events and classes looking like a vast diversity of bodies, abilities, ages, sizes, class backgrounds, practices, races, cultures, gender identities, nationalities and expressions.

This is the world of yoga as unity we can create together.

RECONNECTION

REFLECTION QUESTIONS

What are three actions you can take to shift and interrupt systems of power and oppression?

How can you begin to learn from, listen to and provide platforms for more diverse voices?

Look at the list above and brainstorm more actions you can take as a student, teacher, studio/school owner or director. Which of the actions are you going to take?

If you would like more actions to support you get these Embrace Yoga resources at embraceyogaresources.com.

YOGIS, DEEP LISTENING AND SPEAKING UP

As we practice this path of embodying our yoga as unity, what if you need to bring up the issue of appropriation to someone and don't know how to talk to the person, whether a yoga studio owner or friend?

One of the tools that yoga teaches us is *satya*. *Satya* is the practice of deep listening and loving, compassionate speech (Barkataki, 2018).

Often, we can simply ask someone a question about their intention.

Here, it's important to ask open-ended questions. Open-ended questions are those that invite thought and exploration and don't have a simple "yes" or "no" answer.

For example, you can ask, "Why do you have this statue in the bathroom? What does it mean for you?" in a thoughtful, non-accusatory way. Then, we can listen deeply to the response.

When we listen deeply, we hear another into their truth.

Once you've listened, you can ask, "May I share with you a perspective that you might not have been aware of?" If the person consents, you can share your perspective on how it can be disrespectful or harmful for many people in the yoga tradition to have a manifestation of spiritual wisdom in a place such as the bathroom.

Sometimes, it isn't comfortable to raise conversations like this, even lovingly. In these cases, you can listen deeper into your own intuition. In those moments, the suggestion is to take care of yourself first. To get support and nourishment for your own emotions, grief, anger or suffering.

Finally, it isn't always safe in a place of work or with every person to bring up concerns. Always consider your own or other people's safety when addressing these issues.

R
E
C
O
N
N
E
C
T
I
O
N

HOW TO TALK TO YOUR RELUCTANT FRIENDS OR STUDIOS: PRACTICAL TOOLS FOR ENGAGING IN COURAGEOUS CONVERSATIONS

These guidelines were created to engender safe and brave spaces for challenging and growth-producing conversations. These guidelines have been used for at least a decade in-person, online, in writing and across different cultures, places and spaces to engage challenging, heartfelt and powerful conversations of yoga, equity and justice.

1. BE THOUGHTFUL, UPLIFTING AND KIND

Practice yogic values. For example, *ahimsa* (non-harming and kindness), *satya* (truthfulness), *svadhyaya* (self-inquiry and reflection) and others.

What this might look like concretely:

- Speak from the heart
- Listen deeply from the heart
- Embody respect
- Take risks and lean in to growth

2. STRIVE TO EMBODY AN ETHIC OF MUTUAL GROWTH AND SUPPORT

Respect one another and orient toward growth and support.

3. USE ANTI-OPPRESSIVE METHODS AND MEANS

We are working together to reject the oppressions of colonialism and post-colonialism. As we grapple with complex topics, I invite us to reflect and notice our own positionality, privilege, power and allyship, i.e., belonging to a culture of colonization, colonizer status and/or both.

4. SOLUTIONARY CULTURE

Be solution-oriented. Think of how we can resolve rather than just critique. Take responsibility for our own reactions and feelings. Use call-in vs call-out language. Calling out is an older, power-over model. It often involves using anger, shame or blame to coerce someone into changing their behavior, thoughts or actions. Calling someone in can happen when we ask a kind-hearted question, with the intent to understand, educate or learn.

5. MIND-BODY LEARNING

Check in with body and breath. Self-reflect—process with patience, self-care, self-love and respect. Use "I" statements. Bring a growth mindset, as Dr. Carol Dweck speaks of in her book *Mindset*: "I am not my own or others' mistakes. I'm willing to learn, grow and change and I see that others can, also" (*Mindset*, Dweck).

6. HOLD ROOM FOR MULTIPLE TRUTHS

A decolonizing ethic holds the value of multiple truths and truth as open, available to all, subjective. This is in contrast to the colonial values of truth being objective, scarce and coming from one controlled source. To practice a decolonial inquiry, stay open to both/and possibilities. Be willing to hear someone else's truth as different from yours.

7. CONSIDER CONTEXT

This is big work. Embrace healing as a process. Triggers are normal and natural in this process.

Take care of yourself and others. Own, name, speak when it is right for you (often it is what someone else needs to hear, too). Ask for support: from self, one-on-one, from the group, wider communities and mentors.

RECONNECTION

These guidelines for courageous conversation are offered in the spirit of love, co-creation, connection, decolonial inquiry and evolution. They are not exhaustive, but are part of an ever-evolving process of creation. We are all a critical part of evolving this vital work.

REFLECTION QUESTIONS

- What are some guidelines that would help you feel brave, safe or encouraged enough to have these conversations?

- What is your mindset currently around doing this work?

- What conversations might you need to start with yourself, your community, online or in-person?

TACTICS FOR CHANGE: YOGIS AND HOW TO DO THIS WORK

There are so many ways and levels in which to do this work. We can work from within, create alternative structures, agitate from the outside and more. Here, we will examine some different frameworks for action to create change. Look for where you recognize yourself, where you aspire to be or where you feel resistance.

Across the board, finding where you work best and forming alliances, not enmity, with people who work in different methods and fashions is key.

TACTICS FOR CHANGE

DIRECT SERVICE

Some of us will provide direct service such as creating programs to bring yoga to under-resourced populations. This can be done by educating and creating and building skills.

ART/PROPAGANDA

Some of us will create art, envision, dreaming and manifest visions of what a new and more equitable yoga world will look like, feel like, taste like, smell like and be like. We may create art, media or even propaganda to share this vision.

POLITICAL ORGANIZING

Some of us will work from the inside, within organizations, studios and schools. We may engage with large institutions, companies and structures that are inherently problematic and oppressive. We can bring our newfound tools and values to bear in these environments.

Some of us will lobby, address or advocate for the need for structural and institutional change. We may write letters or articles or call festival organizers, conferences or schools to ask them to do things differently.

COMMUNITY ORGANIZING

Some of us will work with our communities, rallying yoga students, yoga teachers or our wider spheres of influence to address these issues. We may organize large numbers to put pressure on institutions to create change, such as through unionizing or boycotting.

BUILDING ALTERNATIVE INSTITUTIONS

Some of us will work from within alternative structures. For example, we may work to create our own media, our own worker-owned cooperatives, non-profits, funding ventures, trainings, studios or schools.

NONVIOLENT ORGANIZING

Others may work completely from the outside, agitating, disrupting and aiming to dismantle oppressive structures. We may utilize our political, social and community power to address these issues of power and oppression at a systemic level, using many of the above tactics together.

MILITANT REVOLT

Some of us may use more agitating methods, violence, the threat of violence or personal attack to force change. This means is not recommended as a tactic here and is in many ways philosophically out of alignment with yoga practice, but is important to name as it is one of the ways that change occurs.

There may be ways that change occurs that are not named here. The iterations are always evolving. Some of us may work on multiple fronts at once.

Naturally, there can be a tension among these different ways of working, though the aims and values are shared.

Each of us has our particular part to play. Rather than cause further harm by getting caught up in judging or policing the different ways that people do this work, it can be effective to recognize where you operate best and work there.

The goal of addressing separation, reducing oppression and achieving yoga as unity should be the main and unifying principle for our practice, however we act to get there.

REFLECTION QUESTIONS

- Which method(s) of creating change are you most drawn to?

- Which do you dislike or have issues with and why?

- How can you envision working for change while forming alliances with others who are working in different ways?

R
E
C
O
N
N
E
C
T
I
O
N

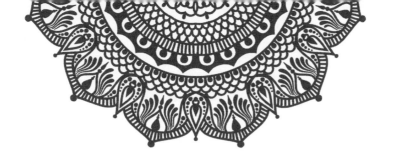

PART 3

EMBRACING WITH REPARATIONS AND INTERSECTIONALITY

"As we build the road, the road builds us."

—A.T. Ariyaratne,
Sri Lankan Activist and Humanitarian

YOGIS AND REPARATIONS

As we continue to do the work of embracing yoga, decolonizing it and appreciating its roots, we aren't only talking about representation, we are also talking about reparations.

WHAT ARE REPARATIONS?

Reparations are a powerful way to address cultural appropriation and are a key practice for yoga practitioners to incorporate today. Reparations involve atoning for what has been stolen and returning many of the benefits, rights and profits of a culture's inheritance to its creators and culture.

Reparations in yoga happen alongside of and in conversation with other movements for reparations such as those for slavery.

We have much to learn from the ongoing leadership of Civil Rights leaders like Patrisse Cullors, Co-Founder of Black Lives Matter:

"Reparations campaigns encompass a wide array of demands. Most commonly, reparations in our contemporary movements are justified by the historical pains and damage caused by European settler colonialism and are proposed in the form of demands for financial restitution, land redistribution, political self-determination, culturally relevant education programs, language recuperation, and the right to return or repatriation," writes Patrisse Cullors (2019), Co-Founder of Black Lives Matter.

The colonial oppression of yoga practitioners in the past and continuing to this day demands the kind of repatriation that Cullors speaks of regarding Black Lives Matter. This critical work of liberation of Black lives is part of what it is to embrace yoga's roots. Our work as yoga practitioners needs to be intersectional and in solidarity and mutuality between the causes of all colonized and oppressed peoples in our work for collective liberation. We as yogis can stand for Black Lives as well as against oppressions based on caste, class, religion or any other form.

WHY REPARATIONS?

Colonial rule and those who benefit from it have profited extensively from the wealth of indigenous resources, labor and knowledge. We must be clear that this isn't just for people of Indian descent, but reparations for all people of color who are harmed by unjust systems of institutional power.

Many yoga studios, schools, businesses, organizations and other power brokers, culture brokers and businesses in Western yoga, in taking a closer look, would see how their use of power has created or contributed to harm in these equations.

Data recently released by renowned economist Utsa Patnaik sifted through nearly two centuries of data on taxes and trade to determine that Britain "drained a total of nearly $45 trillion from India during 1765 and 1938" (2018).

Consider this statistic next to the data from *Yoga Journal* and Yoga Alliance's 2016 IPSOS study that shows yoga is a $16.8 billion-per-year industry. Lululemon, alone, made over $3.19 billion in 2018 (CNBC, 2019).

Given this unfair distribution of wealth and resources, along with staggering economic and labor impacts, we must also consider the cultural, social and spiritual impacts of colonization.

The dehumanization, undermining of tradition and practices, and looting of indigenous ways and beliefs are all the inheritance of modern yoga culture. Not only did Indian trades, labor, jewels and goods fill British coffers, Indian soldiers also fought in the British army, furthering the empire.

This continues today when companies use symbols that are sacred in the yoga tradition, such as *Om* or different deities, as a means of selling more products.

We must speak up so the history of colonial cultural appropriation can shift and change and we can truly embrace the roots of yoga.

R
E
C
O
N
N
E
C
T
I
O
N

WHAT CAN REPARATIONS LOOK LIKE?

Yoga reparations can look many ways. Here are some suggestions:
- Spend your money on those from whom this practice came. Hire South Asian/Desi yoga teachers.
- Hire and consult with BIPOC race equity and yoga teachers.
- Learn and practice the full expanse of what yoga can be.
- Buy books written by South Asian authors.
- Donate money to organizations doing humanitarian work in India or

to organizations dedicated to the preservation of the yoga tradition within India.

You can also research your own ideas for reparations and/or see the Resource List at the end of this book.

REFLECTION QUESTIONS

⊛ What questions or concerns do you have about giving yoga reparations?

⊛ How can you give yoga reparations?

⊛ Who are you going to uplift?

YOGIS AND INTERSECTIONALITY

"Being a Desi yogi means to me loving and fighting for all our culture has offered to the world and celebrating with ritual and reflection."

—Susanna Barkataki

The term 'intersectionality' was coined by scholar and writer Kimberlé Crenshaw (1989). It refers to how categories like race, class, gender, sexuality and ability are interconnected and work together to affect our individual and collective experiences. The concept also explains how these categories correlate to different, yet connected, systems of oppression, power and privilege.

"Intersectionality is a lens through which you can see where power comes and collides, where it interlocks and intersects. It's not simply that there's a race problem here, a gender problem here, and a class or LBGTQ problem there. Many times that framework erases what happens to people who are subject to all of these things" (Crenshaw, 2017).

In yoga today, we must consider intersectionality and move beyond inclusion. We can find ever-evolving ways to learn, embrace and celebrate yoga history. In addition to inclusion, we must expand yoga norms and celebrate yoga history and diversity.

If we are living in a culture that upholds whiteness and perpetuates anti-blackness, our work to address these issues must be intersectional. For many people of color who are reclaiming their rightful heritage of body movement and healing, yoga and other movement forms are a pathway to reclamation. South Asians can stand alongside Black, Brown and other people of color in reclaiming our practices and uplifting one another in leadership in these spaces.

Additionally, we need to address the fundamentalist violence that is being enacted in yoga's name in India. The Hindu Indian government is

RECONNECTION

excluding ethnic and religious minorities from civil events, citizenship, registries and other forms of economic and legal violence. It is intersectional to love yoga but not love or support the exclusion and fundamentalism it is being misused to justify.

It is important for us to know this context in the West as the homeland of yoga herself is struggling.

Again, this doesn't mean don't practice or teach if you aren't Indian. It does mean lifting up your BIPOC, South Asian and Indian counterparts.

REFLECTION QUESTIONS

- What is intersectionality in your own words?

- Instead of allowing the status quo to amplify, what can you do to learn the history, uplift teachers of color and focus on philosophy, ethics and other aspects of yoga?

- Can we live as if we are all connected? Acknowledging that we already are, how might we express this?

RECONNECTION

YOGIS AND CREATIVITY

Engaging in practicing yoga as liberation, avoiding appropriation and acting for equity is inherently creative.

As we do the work of embracing yoga as unity it can also feel like creative play. We are sharing the tools of yoga so everyone can become free. We can live yoga as unity, not denying our differences, but celebrating our unique humanity, practicing inclusion and diversity to achieve equity.

Creativity is enlivened by commitment to action. (And then keep doing it!) Commit to and act on these truths. Your awareness is powerful when paired with action.

Here are a few ways to bring creativity-in-action alive:
- Creativity comes alive in our daily actions—pay attention to them.
- Take small, consistent steps.
- Do not pigeonhole this work as an add-on to your practice.
- Allow radical inclusivity to be something you embody. Something you are.
- Ask, "What am I doing that may create more separation?"
- Then, "How can I embody inclusivity and union?"

You don't need to be perfect. Remember: Perfectionism is a tool of white supremacy and we are undoing white-supremacy thinking.

Though we are not aiming for perfection, we *are* aiming for endurance and consistency. You must try, and fall and get up and try again. It's about embodying a kind of devotion to the heart of yoga, the heart of our practice.

Creativity in our practice involves tuning in to our own ancestral lineage. Listening deeply to the stirrings, calls and questions that arise within. Giving time, space and voice to ancestral wisdom. We each have lineages. We each have stories of resilience and suffering in our lines. We can learn from these stories, felt, intuited, researched, as well as told.

Creativity is going within our own experience so deeply that we bring alive the authentic and sacred parts of ourselves.

RECONNECTION

REFLECTION QUESTIONS

- How does creativity help support us in not appropriating?

- How can you explore and embody creativity in your journey of unity?

- What do you commit to take forward to embrace the roots and spirit of yoga?

RECONNECTION

YOGIS AND YOUR VITAL VOICE

In this work of embracing yoga, your voice is needed.

We are the ones who are responsible for preserving the heart and soul of this powerful practice for future generations; for ensuring that a full spectrum of yoga is preserved and shared.

You embrace yoga by going deep into the heart of yogic practice. Listen deeply, practice *ahimsa*. Non-harming. And *satya*. Truth-telling. *Satya* isn't just speaking, it's listening in such a way that truth emerges.

This is the lesser-known and lesser-taught aspect of *satya*. The type of deep listening that invites radical, authentic truths to emerge. *Satya* isn't just about your own voice, it's about all of our voices. It's about the voices we don't hear. It's about the voices we've all but lost.

Satya is about listening in a way that the suppressed truths of a person or situation are invited to come to light. *Satya* is speaking truth to power. *Satya* is allowing the truth of yoga as union to speak to us. To come through us.

We can let yoga as union come through us and speak through us.

This takes all of us and our full truth. We are telling all of our truths here. Our messy, beautiful, personal, mythic, powerful resonant truths.

Explore the heart of your *satya*. Your truth.

REFLECTION QUESTIONS

⚜ What truths are you listening into being?

⚜ What or whose truths in yoga are you going to listen to more deeply?

⚜ What truths are you going to speak aloud or amplify?

VI

LIBERATION

"Of all the instruments of emancipation, Love is supreme."

—Sri Adi Shankaracharya

PART 1

YOGIS AND UNITY

*"The ideal is to live in the world in
full awareness of life's unity."*

—Eknath Easwaran

Inherent in the practice of yoga is the work of creating unity. Unity of the small self with the greater self. Unity of each individual with the greater whole. As we have discussed, yoga, *yuj*, to yoke, is defined as unity. We move toward overcoming separation when we practice yoga as unity.

We must lean back, embrace roots and dismantle appropriation, to move forward.

As we embrace yoga's roots as well as our own, we are untangling the roots of colonization and empire, the intertwined causes of separation such as all the isms—racism, sexism, ableism, etc.—as ways to create inner and outer transformation.

We can decolonize and embrace our practice by looking back to the roots and heart of yoga as we practice forward. There are specific tools for this that we can learn from the tradition itself. With yoga, unity is right here. It's always within.

The beauty is that everyone can connect to it—we all have this within us. No one need be left out. It is available to all. Just ask and yoga will speak to you.

If we want yoga, we cannot run from what it means to truly practice yoga. Yoga is union. If we can breathe, we can do yoga. If we can feel, we represent liberation. And when we breathe together, we all get a little more free.

Breathe in this future with me.
Breathe out and let's make it happen together.

FROM SEPARATION TO LIBERATION

Yoga has always had liberation as its aim.

Liberation has multiple meanings. Often in its early usage in yogic texts as *kaivalya* it is referring to freedom from illusion of the cycle of suffering that humans experience. Liberation is the awareness of our true nature as always already interconnected to everything else. It is the realization of no separation between oneself and others.

Early yoga practitioners were aiming at finding liberation from suffering, from a small sense of self, from the confines of this world (Mallinson and Singleton, 2017).

In Patanjali's Yoga Sutras it is described this way:

> puruṣa-artha-śūnyānāṁ guṇānāṁ-pratiprasavaḥ kaivalyaṁ
> svarūpa-pratiṣṭhā vā citiśaktiriti Yoga Sutra 4.34

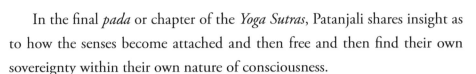

In the final *pada* or chapter of the *Yoga Sutras*, Patanjali shares insight as to how the senses become attached and then free and then find their own sovereignty within their own nature of consciousness.

Often this pursuit of liberation led to detaching from the senses to become aware of the absolute experience of self in the early yogic context.

In the West, we often take the opposite view. Liberation is seen as an individualistic expression of self where our desires run rampant. This is not the kind of freedom that yoga promises.

Our current context of liberation, such as the definition and understanding growing out of the civil rights movement in the United States in the 1950s and 1960's, can also mean freedom from all constraints of oppression and discrimination.

This work of embracing yoga's roots respects multiple contexts for liberation.

The work of detatching from the senses and stories we bring to the world can help us find liberation for ourselves and others.

Instead of ignoring or pretending separation doesn't exist, we've now explored and deepened your understanding of the causes of separation. We've built your skills up to reflect on your part. And we do all of this work so we can move toward true unity.

The solution to the problem of separation is in the path of yoga itself. Here, within the yogic path, we have our roadmap for personal and social transformation, for a revolution within and without.

Yoga is a bridge and a way to connect us to ourselves and to one another. In this next section, we will begin to listen to yoga's roots as our pathway out of separation and towards liberation.

L
I
B
E
R
A
T
I
O
N

REFLECTION QUESTIONS

⚜ Has yoga helped you feel more connected to yourself and others? Where has yoga led to liberation for you personally?

⚜ Has yoga led to liberation for you beyond yourself—perhaps in your family, community or other places around you?

⚜ What does personal liberation have to do with collective liberation?

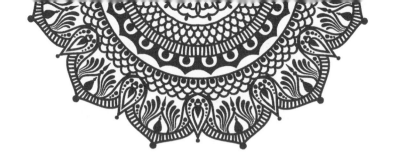

PART 2

YOGA ETHICS IN ACTION FOR LIBERATION

"The success of yoga does not lie in the ability to perform postures but in how it positively changes the way we live our lives and our relationships."

—T.K.V. DESIKACHAR

YOU CAN EMBRACE YOGA AND FIND PERSONAL AND COLLECTIVE LIBERA-tion by going deep into the heart of yogic practice. By looking at the essence of this practice, we find ways to reclaim and honor it. When you practice yoga ethics, you make a strong commitment for love, for peace, for justice and for care of ourselves, each other, all beings and the world.

Here are my interpretations of *Patanjali's* eight limbs from book 1 of the *Yoga Sutras*. I utilized the teachings of Satchidananda (2012) as well as Iyengar (1989) as sources for these interpretations.

YOGA ETHICS AND THE EIGHT-LIMBED PATH

1. *Yamas*—Outer, ethical codes
2. *Niyamas*—Inner, personal transformation codes
3. *Asana*—Physical practice
4. *Pranayama*—Breathwork
5. *Pratyahara*—Focus
6. *Dharana*—Mindfulness
7. *Dhyana*—Meditation
8. *Samadhi*—Bliss

THE YAMA

The *yama*, or as they are referred to colloquially in the West, the *yamas*, are ethical guidelines for action.

Viveka, or wise discernment, is a deep yogic practice of yogic ethics that invites you to be engaged in the world. Yoga is not a passive practice. Nor is it a practice to put down when you roll up your yoga mat. Yoga is, truly, an engaged social justice practice. These versions of the *yamas* and *niyamas* are written to invite engagement through every aspect of life and, as such, are written as commitments and affirmations. These interpretations are inspired by Sri Swami Satchidananda and Shankaracharya's interpretations of *Patanjali's Yoga Sutras*.

The *yama* and *niyama* can represent a yogic vision for a global yoga practice, lifestyle and ethic. They are a concrete expression of the practice and teachings of yoga and the Eight-Limbed Path. Living by them can create transformation, healing and happiness for ourselves and the world. Practicing the limbs of yoga, we follow our inner guidance to personal, emotional, physical and spiritual growth. With them, we can cultivate a life of truth, compassion, generosity and peace.

The *Yama* are outer, ethical codes and can guide us in how we relate to others.

LIBERATION

AHIMSA—is practicing non-violence and non-harming to yourself, people, animals and the environment. Practice kindness above all. Practicing *ahimsa*, I cultivate openness and non-discrimination toward myself and others. I am nonviolent toward myself, have regard for all beings to transform suffering in myself and in the world.

SATYA—is practicing honesty in thought, word or deed. I practice truthful thinking, speech and action in order to promote reconciliation and peace in myself and among others. I listen deeply to hear others into their own truths. I use open communication and do my best to resolve all conflicts. I know words can create happiness or suffering so I use my words and my listening to inspire joy, confidence and positivity.

ASTEYA—is practicing with the awareness that I have everything I need right here, inside of myself. I embody non-stealing, embracing what belongs to others and celebrating what we have. A sense of abundance gives rise to confidence that I have what I need. I cultivate a deep satisfaction with life.

BRAHMACHARYA—is energy management, practicing to embrace and respect all life energy including breath, sexual energy and life force. I know our energy is sacred, so I respect it and cherish it. I manage my energy to preserve positive and uplifting experiences for myself and others. I honor my own and others' boundaries.

APARIGRAHA—is practicing non-grasping. Release of craving and aversion. I allow and let go. I know all things will change. Impermanence is a part of life. This allows me a greater freedom from attachment and helps me let go of expectations. I accept that change is constant, everything is temporary, and from this I find freedom. I am committed to cultivating the insight of interbeing and compassion.

THE NIYAMA

The *niyama* or as they are called colloquially in the West, the *niyamas*, are inner, personal codes for living a soulful and spiritual yogic life.

SAUCHA—In practicing *saucha*, I maintain clear and pure mind, body and surroundings. I know my environment and what I consume reflects in my consciousness and I live accordingly. I maintain a clean household, body, speech and actions. If needed, I create space and time for purification and clearing out what no longer serves my highest good.

SANTOSHA—I practice *santosha* by aiming to cultivate happiness in as many moments as possible. I turn my mind toward gratitude to nourish contentment. I grow and learn from the events in my life. I strive to have a positive outlook and learn from and cultivate peace. I take pleasure in the present moment. I do what I love and enjoy myself.

TAPAS—I practice *tapas* by committing to my practice with discipline and focus. I harness yogic discipline for the power of good. I use the fire within to change myself for the better. I cultivate and find enthusiasm for daily spiritual practice. I apply consistent effort to maintaining wellness with a steady application of energy. I balance discipline and devotion.

SVHADYAYA—I explore myself and know through understanding myself that I come to understand all. I study my Self. I observe my actions and inquire within with curiosity and non-judgment. I stay attentive to what needs to be let go and what needs care and nourishment.

ISHVARA PRANIDHANA—I practice *ishvara pranidhana* by dedicating myself to divine texts and practices, being aware of the interconnection of all beings, and honoring energies greater than myself. I practice yoga as unity. I am in devotion to the divine as I see and understand it. I experience life as meaningful. I am devoted to higher purpose, in service to Spirit and live a good life for myself and others. I know in connecting to one I am connected to all.

Practicing with these ethical foundations is a lifelong journey toward personal and social transformation. It begins here and now with simple steps.

L
I
B
E
R
A
T
I
O
N

REFLECTION QUESTIONS

⚬ Which of the *yamas* are you working to incorporate in your life right now?

⚬ Which of the *niyamas* are you working to incorporate in your life right now?

⚬ How can practicing yoga ethics help you embrace yoga's roots?

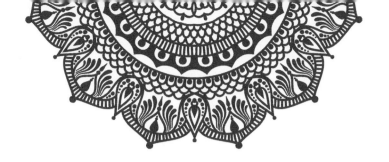

PART 3

HOW TO STRUCTURE AN ASANA CLASS TO EMBRACE YOGA'S ROOTS

"Sthira Sukham Asanam"

—Patanjali Yoga Sutra 2.46

FRAMEWORK FOR AN ASANA CLASS TO EMBRACE YOGA'S ROOTS

Living a yogic lifestyle is a great part of teaching yoga in a respectful way. Incorporating the deeper philosophical aspects of yoga—such as *dharana* (mindful focus), *dhyana* (meditation) and ethics such as the *yamas* and *niyamas*—in your life is a helpful and necessary prerequisite for teaching *asana* to others.

This outline assumes you are practicing with a richer understanding of what yoga is. It does not assume you have perfected this inquiry, as the idea is that we are all growing and evolving in our studentship.

BEFORE BEGINNING CLASS

Set the container for yourself. Meditate, pray, set your intention. In your way, ground yourself in the widened awareness of the present moment and a sense of unity and connection that yoga offers us.

PREPARE THE SPACE

In yoga, all actions are sacred. Cleaning and preparing the space is part of your practice. From sweeping the floor to laying out props for your students, every action you do can be one of devotion.

GREETING YOUR CLASS

Find a way that works for you personally to greet your students. Perhaps you welcome them each by name, ask how they are doing, or take a moment of personal connection with each person. This would be a beautiful place to say *namaste*, if you like to incorporate Sanskrit, as it is a traditional way of greeting one another used in South Asia.

LAND AND SPIRITUAL LINEAGE ACKNOWLEDGMENT: EMBRACE THE ROOTS OF YOGA

Just as you may do a land acknowledgment to honor the land you are teaching and practicing on and all those who live there, as we will describe below, do a spiritual lineage acknowledgment. Open your practice by countering the erasure of thousands of years of codification and development of yoga science by Indians and other Asian and African people by acknowledging the roots of the practice. Always offer a spiritual lineage acknowledgment at the start of your yoga practice, workshop or event.

BEGINNING YOUR CLASS

Rather than diving in with *asana*, consider beginning with *dharana* (mindful focus) or *dhyana* (meditation). The aim of yoga *asana* practice is to steady the mind for meditation and focus. By guiding students in this way, perhaps through a short guided meditation or through a sensory-based attention activity, you are helping direct them toward a more engaged yoga practice.

INVITE STUDENTS TO EXPLORE YOGA BEYOND THE MAT BY INCLUDING YOGA PHILOSOPHY

Instead of including yoga philosophy as an afterthought or an add-on, ensure that it is an integral part of your class.

Perhaps you may tie in a short explanation of a theme from yoga philosophy that you are personally working on in-depth to help the class see more of what is possible in yoga.

For example, you could tie in the theme of *ahimsa* when describing how the goal of the practice isn't perfection, or doing what someone else is doing or even what they did last week or last year, but instead it's experiencing the shape they are in right here and now, with compassion for themselves rather than competition.

When we guide students by invoking yoga philosophy, we are guiding them to the present moment of their experience, right here and now.

SETTING THE SANKALPA

When inviting students to set an intention for class, you can refer them to yoga philosophy. For example, you can mention they are exploring their own *satya*, or truth, and engaging in *vichara* and *svadhyaya* as they self-reflect.

L
I
B
E
R
A
T
I
O
N

IF YOU TEACH ASANA CLASS

Remember, teaching *asana* is not a prerequisite for teaching yoga. Your class can focus entirely on yoga philosophy, meditation, mindfulness or breath. Though teaching *asana* is not the only way to teach yoga, *asanas* are here to support us in moving toward more mindfulness. As such, ensure as you teach that you are utilizing *asana* and not forgetting about pointing students to deeper states of engagement and connection. From the beginning, you can let students know they are the leaders and you, as their teacher, are the guide. This focus on the practitioner and their own deepening awareness and connection to their own truth and wisdom is at the heart of yogic practice.

Guide students into present-moment inquiry in each *asana*. As they move into and breathe into each shape, provide guidance to remind them to come back to their own awareness of self in each moment.

FOCUS ON THE BREATH

Personal study and practice of *pranayama* (breath practice) is an important part of yoga. Whether you directly teach *pranayama* or not, you can always remind and guide your students to come back to taking full, deep breaths in each shape they are in or moving through.

FOCUS ON BENEFITS, NOT ACCOMPLISHMENTS

Focus on the benefits for the *asana* shapes. Whether someone is practicing a shape on the ground, a chair or standing, the benefit of the *asana* should be similar. The goal is not physical attainment or standardization of the shape, but presence and peace of mind. Cue in such a way as to bring students into more presence and peace.

END WITH DHARANA

When appropriate, end with meditation. Guiding students to meditate is in line with the original aims of yoga practice. Learn to guide meditation for yoga *asana* classes. You can guide students in 5 to 10 minutes of *dharana* practice before or after *savasana.* Take time in meditation to let the benefits of the practice settle and integrate.

CLOSING CLASS

As you close your class, thank your students.

Consider dedicating the practice to something greater than all of you, or to their highest intentions.

LAND AND SPIRITUAL LINEAGE ACKNOWLEDGEMENT: HOW TO OPEN YOUR ASANA PRACTICE TO EMBRACE YOGA'S ROOTS

LAND ACKNOWLEDGMENT AND CONTEXT

Land acknowledgment is a necessary part of living as settler colonials on land to which we are not indigenous.

A land acknowledgment is a formal statement that recognizes, names and situates Indigenous Peoples as traditional stewards of the land you are on and respects the relationship between them and their traditional land.

When we do not do land acknowledgments, we erase indigenous presence, history and disenfranchisement.

According to the Department of Arts and Agriculture (U.S.D.A.C., 2019):

> "Acknowledgment is a simple, powerful way of showing respect and a step toward correcting the stories and practices

L
I
B
E
R
A
T
I
O
N

that erase Indigenous people's history and culture and toward inviting and honoring the truth. Imagine this practice widely adopted: imagine cultural venues, classrooms, conference settings, acknowledging traditional lands. Millions would be exposed—many for the first time—to the names of the traditional Indigenous inhabitants of the lands they are on, inspiring them to ongoing awareness and action."

HOW TO DO A LAND ACKNOWLEDGMENT

To do a land acknowledgment begin by finding out whose land you are on. Speak the names of people and places. Address whether the territory you are on is ceded or unceded land. There may be native folks who are working to regain sovereignty over the land you are on.

You can say, something like, "I am here on un-ceded Seminole land."

Then, ideally, for an event you invite in someone from the First Nations people or tribe to do a land acknowledgment and lead an opening to the space you are creating.

Invite respectfully. When you invite folks in it is important to do it respectfully. To build relationships and plan to invite them to attend your event for free as VIP guests. It is also important to honor the time and wisdom of the leaders by offering a stipend, payment, honorarium or asking what they would wish to receive in exchange for giving of their time, experience and hard won knowledge.

Just as it is important to honor the land we are on and people it is from, it is important in a yoga context to honor the spiritual lineage of the practice.

SPIRITUAL LINEAGE ACKNOWLEDGMENT IN YOGA

A spiritual lineage acknowledgment honors the lineage, indigenous wisdom and heritage of the practice of yoga.

L
I
B
E
R
A
T
I
O
N

Just as you may do a land acknowledgment, at the beginning of any yoga-related class, workshop, training, conference or in-person or online event, you should do a spiritual lineage acknowledgment.

The spiritual lineage acknowledgment should become protocol and policy in yoga contexts alongside land acknowledgments.

We need to each be performing land acknowledgments as well as spiritual lineage acknowledgments.

When doing a Spiritual Lineage Acknowledgment, no one ever has to name an abuser in the name of embracing yoga's roots. There have been many cases of abuse within different spiritual lineages including within many yoga lineages. In no way does doing a Spiritual Lineage Acknowledgment mean you need to name or honor a teacher or teachers who have been abusive. You can address and honor spiritual lineage by saying something like, "I appreciate the spiritual seekers and teachers from India who developed and codified this practice. . ." without needing to name an abusive teacher. More on this topic is shared in the the important work of Karen Rain, Jubilee Cook as well as other #MeToo Yoga activists and in the book *Embodied Resilience through Yoga: 30 Mindful Essays About Finding Empowerment After Addiction, Trauma, Grief, and Loss.*

As part of embracing the roots of yoga we ask that all individuals and organizations in spaces from yoga classes to workshops, in all open public events in person or online, acknowledge the traditional South Asian originators of the rich spiritual tradition of yoga. By doing this you go a long way towards inviting in a more respectful connection to the practice.

As we embrace yoga's roots we need to look with an intersectional lens. In practicing a lineage acknowledgment, one does not need to name predatory, harmful or violent teachers within a tradition. Acknowledging the roots of the tradition can go further back to speak of the Indian, or Brown and Black teachers or practitioners who gave rise to this practice.

LIBERATION

HOW TO DO A SPIRITUAL LINEAGE ACKNOWLEDGMENT

The steps for doing a spiritual lineage acknowledgment are simple and important.

1. Name the culture and people from whom yoga comes, and where it was organized, practiced and codified: India.

2. Speak your teacher(s) by name. Explore the lineage of your own teaching and the teachers of your teachers. Name them and bring them into the room.

3. Remind students that they are in a context of spiritual practice and learning. Invite them to practice gratitude for this teaching that comes down to us through space and time from the practitioners of yoga in the past.

4. Go to every effort possible to invite in the people from whom this practice comes. When possible, invite indigenous South Asian or Desi stewards to lead this spiritual acknowledgment. Follow the guidelines above to invite respectfully. Practice honoring and re-spectful protocol when engaging with experts and practitioners from within these wisdom traditions. If it is not possible to bring in a representative you can still do steps 1, 2 and 3.

For example, you could begin your yoga class by saying,

> "I want to begin by embracing the roots of the sacred tradi-tion of yoga, and all of the yogis, from India, from *Shiva* to *Patanjali*, down through time and space, who have practiced and taught so that we can benefit today. I thank my teachers *Shankarji* and *Kabirji* and all of our teachers. I honor every single teacher who has brought us here today."

We ask that all individuals and organizations hosting yoga-related events begin with acknowledgment of the traditional and indigenous practitioners and teachers of this practice in a spiritual lineage acknowledgment.

LIBERATION

Always offer a spiritual lineage acknowledgment at the start of your yoga practice, workshop or event.

Opening with Spiritual Lineage Acknowledgment is how we can shift each class, workshop, training and event to more Embrace the Roots of Yoga.

NAMASTE AND HOW TO CLOSE AN ASANA PRACTICE THAT EMBRACES YOGA'S ROOTS

Do you say *Namaste* when you close your yoga *asana* class and why?

Are you embracing the culture and pronouncing it correctly?

Are you attached to it? If so, why?

Is there another way to convey the same resonance, beauty, wisdom?

Namaste has become a signifier of the end of a yoga class. It has a beautiful meaning.

Namaste has the connotation of reverence, adoration, saluting and bowing. It also has within it the reference to the second person—to you. There is no reference to I as in—I bow to you—or I salute you. *Namaste* is focused on the person being greeted and saluted.

I find this so powerful, as I often do when studying the intricacies and layers of Sanskrit's meaning, because the I or ego is completely absent. To me, this enlivens *how* in *namaste*, the energy, or essence of revering, bowing and adoring is all there is.

Namaste is a state or way of being. And perhaps as diaphanous and aspirational a goal as yoga itself. Should you use *namaste* to end class? Let's explore.

In this inquiry, I aim here, as I often do, to not give absolute answers but to ask you questions to inspire the yogic practice of *Vichāra*—critical thinking.

In my own personal experience living in India and with my elders and family here in the U.S., "*Namaste*" or "*Namaskar*" is said when I meet and greet an elder. Not when I leave.

It feels rather formal. It feels strange and culturally off to say it at the end of class for me personally. Though I certainly have done it. I usually don't now.

Why not? I notice that it's become a signifier, a glamorizing of Eastern culture. To use *"Namaste"* telegraphs our positionality as a teacher. Something like using the exoticism of a foreign word connotes "I, the wise yoga teacher, am now importing some wisdom to you." Or sometimes, when we want to signal "class is over, y'all can go"—in so many spiritual-sounding words—it's an easy way to get students out the door.

Also, though I've often been corrected by popular Western yoga teachers, it's actually pronounced more like "na-muh-steh," with the emphasis on the second syllable, by my Indian family and teachers.

Not "nam-ah-staaay" with the emphasis on the third syllable, like we often hear incorrectly sing-songed at the end of yoga classes.

The alternative to appropriation is often creativity.

Can we get creative on how we may convey the same inspirational and spiritual sentiment in an appropriate way?

I invite and challenge both myself and you to get creative. Now let me be clear. You don't have to change anything.

This is an invitation to explore how you might creatively convey the feeling + message you wish to in your voice!

You can close with a thank-you, or there are many other options. You can find a list of sixty-plus ways to end your yoga class on my website here: www.susannabarkataki.com/post/namaste.

Remember, traditionally, *namaste* is said at the beginning of a meeting with another highly respected person, not at the end.

You can close with other traditional closings such as *Om, Shanti, Shanti, Shanti.*

Om, peace, peace, peace. Or with a thank-you. Or develop your own closing to your class.

REFLECTION QUESTIONS

- What elements of yoga philosophy do you want to learn more about and practice?

- What lesser-known practices from the yoga tradition can you bring into your class?

- How can you prepare for your class in a more respectful, honoring and embracing way?

APPLICATIONS

- How can you open your class in a way that embraces yoga's roots?

- How can you teach your class in a way that embraces yoga's roots?

- How can you close your class in a way that embraces yoga's roots?

LIBERATION

YOGA BEYOND ASANA: WHAT DOES A WORLD OF EMBRACING YOGA LOOK LIKE?

"There is no power equal to yoga."

—*The Mahabharata* 12.304.2ab

Yoga is a subtle science that focuses on bringing harmony between mind and body. There are many techniques that make up this science that extend far beyond *asana*.

The word 'yoga' has many meanings throughout its use in early pre-Vedic and Vedic times. In fact, this word has perhaps more meanings than any other word in Sanskrit. What most of the codification of yoga has in common is a description of yoga as a path to liberation from the small self to join with a larger, unified sense of oneness (Mallinson, Singleton, 2017).

Yoga does not belong to one specific religion, though it has developed alongside and influenced many. Yoga is seen by many "a technology for inner wellbeing," according to Dr. Ishwar V. Basavaraddi, Director of India's Ministry of Public Affairs, and anyone who practices yoga with involvement can reap its benefits, irrespective of one's faith, ethnicity or culture.

There are various schools of yoga within the tradition, some formal guru-*parampara* (guru lineage teacher to student) and some practical schools, such as *Jnana* (knowledge), *Bhakti* (devotion), *Karma* (action), *Raja* (Kingly) and so on. Each school has its own principles and practices leading to their own understanding of yoga.

Given this rich history, there are many ways to embrace yoga's roots that fall within the tradition. When we embrace yoga, we practice in a way that shares the fullness of a well-rounded yoga practice. We develop a deep relationship to all of the eight limbs of yoga, as well as other yogic practices such as *vichara* (self-inquiry), *tapas* (discipline and austerity practices), *band-*

has and *mudras* (energy locks), *drishti* (steadiness of the gaze) and *mantra* (repetition of sound) (Mallinson, Singleton, 2017).

If we are serious about embracing yoga's roots, it is important for us to develop a yoga practice that goes beyond *asana*. We can develop this practice through word-of-mouth from a traditioned or lineaged teacher, through reading sacred or yogic texts, through study and through practice.

DEEPENING YOGA SADHANA

There are many Yoga *Sadhana* (yoga practices) in addition to the eightfold path that we often study within *Patanjali's Yoga Sutras*. These eight pillars are important, and we can add to them more practices inherent in yoga. It is beyond the scope of this text to give a full explanation of each of these practices. Also consider that, in my *Hatha* yoga tradition, I have been taught that many of them must be imparted in-person by a trained teacher and practitioner.

What follows is an explanation for clarification, and to invite you to deepen your practice through study, reading, practice and all means available to you.

Vichara (self-inquiry)—*Vichara* practice is done through reflection, self-observation and critique of oneself.

Tapas (discipline and austerity practices)—*Tapas* is often translated as burning fire. Traditionally, it is considered to be the practices we do that are the hardest and that burn away impurities in the mind and body.

Pranayama (expansion of vital life force through the breath)—*Pranayama* is the control or movement of breath and life force through the body. Inhalation, retention of the breath in, exhalation and retention of the breath out are all steps in the use of this yogic method. There are many different *pranayama* techniques with various benefits, which require instruction from a trained teacher.

Bandhas and *Mudras* (energy locks)—*Bandhas* and *mudras* are tools that aid in controlling the mind and body. *Bandhas* refer to specific "locks" at

LIBERATION

the root, center and throat. *Mudras* refer to seals or gestures made with the hands, legs or the whole body. Both practices work on the subtle, as well as gross body.

Drishti (steadiness of the gaze)—The practice of focusing the gaze, whether with eyes open, closed, or gaze soft allows the inner eye to strengthen and balance to grow.

Mantra (repetition of sound)—*Mantra* is the repetition of sacred sound, whether aloud, whispered or silently in the mind. *Mantra* is a support for the mind. *Mantra* can be practiced with *mala* beads, in which case, it is called *japa* practice. One practices moving one bead per sound of the *mantra*.

Samadhi / Samyama—*Samyama* is the combined practice of *dharana* (mindfulness), *dhyana* (concentration) and *samadhi* (bliss), otherwise known as insight states accessible during meditation. *Samyama* is the practice of these experiences combined. Yoga *Sadhana* (practice) is the deepening of these many and varied practices.

Yoga is a lifelong path of exploration and study.

My sincere wish is that you have broadened your understanding of what it is to practice yoga beyond the surface and now have many concrete and inspiring considerations for taking the practice off the mat and into your life.

I look forward to your continued journey to practice and embrace yoga's roots.

REFLECTION QUESTIONS

- Where may my practice be causing separation?

- Am I embracing yoga's authentic roots and my own authentic cultural connection and values?

- Which yogic practice can I do more to create connection?

LIBERATION

VII

HOW TO CONTINUE
THIS WORK

"There is no yoga without justice. There is no peace without yoga. No justice, no peace."

— Susanna Barkataki

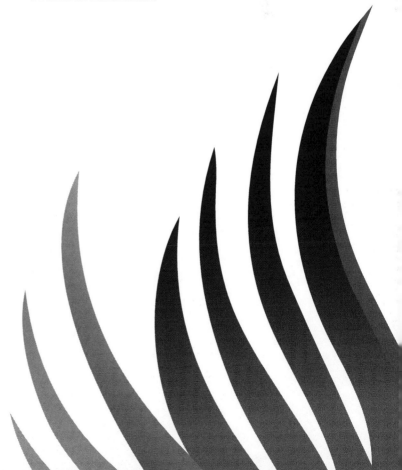

HOW DO I CONTINUE THIS WORK?

Yoga is here for us to cultivate power and transcend our very limitations, personally and socially. Not to create more separation but as a way to connect, dissolving separation within and without.

We can live an authentic, embodied yoga practice for equity and spiritual fulfillment. Together, we can lean back on authentic yoga culture as a vessel for shaping change now.

We can allow yoga to speak to us and through us as vessels of transformation.

The work of deepening in yoga can take a lifetime. My teacher used to joke that it could take many lifetimes!

Know that deepening in this work takes practice. It takes embodying our yoga and applying critical thinking in each new circumstance. If I could have written a book that listed 365 definitive steps to take to not culturally appropriate, I would have. However, this work of honoring and not appropriating yoga isn't so simple. It takes critical thinking and deep, embodied practice to embrace yoga's roots.

This work is ongoing and iterative. There is beauty here in the process. We are each necessary parts in the work of honoring rather than appropriating yoga. It doesn't end.

Here are some resources and suggestions for things you can do to keep the work going. At different times, different practices may resonate. Listen. Uplift. Educate. Agitate. And keep going.

REFLECT AND PRACTICE
THE EMBRACE YOGA FRAMEWORK

The Embrace Yoga Framework involves honoring the roots of the practice. A key way to do this is to always offer a spiritual lineage acknowledgment at the start of your yoga practice, workshop or event.

Invite in indigenous stewards to lead this spiritual acknowledgment.

Ask yourself questions from the Embrace Yoga's Roots framework to see if you are embracing yoga.

1. Is it causing separation? Is it unsafe? Harmful? Safe? Kind?
2. Am I embracing roots? Consider yoga's roots, as well as your own.
3. Does it create connection—to yourself, to others, for a group?
4. Does it lead to liberation? Does it make you more mindful, free, peaceful, powerful or calm?

This work is continually about relationship and willingness to connect. To learn. To try. To converse and discuss across differences.

We are here together. To grow. To learn. To do better. To embrace yoga.

By listening and applying this framework to your own actions and practice, you will go far toward embracing yoga.

PRIVILEGE/TARGET T-CHART

On this T-Chart, brainstorm the areas where you hold privilege or target identities. For example, I will demonstrate some of mine below.

Privilege Identities I Hold (Susanna Barkataki)	Target Identities I Hold (Susanna Barkataki)
Educational privilege (college and master's degree) Mixed/Lighter-skinned privilege Cisgender Heterosexual passing	Immigrant Woman BIPOC with Brown skin Trauma survivor Disabled Queer

Privilege Identities You Hold	Target Identities You Hold

ANTI-WHITE-SUPREMACY
EMBRACE YOGA COMMITMENTS

Here are mine. Add to these or create your own.

Instead of uniqueness, highlight community.

Instead of focusing on perfecting posture, focus on processing and feeling within a shape.

Offer self and others incremental growth that supports where someone is at.

Instead of yoga celebrities, create and uplift communities.

Instead of obsession with the body, focus on obsession of the heart, service, intuition and spiritual realization and freedom.

Instead of frontlining more white yoga teachers or tokenizing POC, invite, uplift and provide platforms for multiple teachers of color in every yoga space.

Instead of solely focusing on physicality, focus on yoga philosophy, ethics and spirituality.

Instead of perfectionism, focus our culture on progress, process and growth as benchmarks for success.

Provide platforms for many different voices and experiences (and do not tokenize the one POC teacher in the process).

Instead of participating and furthering dominant norms, help make yoga norms open-source; celebrate multiple narratives and pluralistic representation.

Being willing to research the historical and cultural context of a ritual or practice before adopting it.

Being willing to self-inquire: Does this belong in my studio, on my body, in my home?

Quote, cite and give respect to the origins of the practice wherever possible.

If you have been invited to speak on a yoga panel, summit, conference, festival, ask, "Who else has been invited to speak?" to impel equal representation.

As you continue to practice, come back to your Embrace Yoga's Roots framework to guide you.

By listening, learning and continuing to apply this framework to your own actions and practice, you will go far toward embracing yoga.

RESOURCES TO RESEARCH / LEARN FROM / DONATE TO

As part of this Embrace Yoga's Roots movement, donations are made to South Asian justice organizations in South Asia and in diaspora abroad as well as to organizations in support of Black Lives, Dalit Equity and Indigenous First Nations justice.

Reparations are long overdue and no end to this need is in sight. Thus, donations and support are always welcome if you are able and want to send your own gifts to any of the reparations organizations we share here as part of your commitment to embracing yoga's roots.

As the work evolves and grows, this list will always evolve, change and grow. The most current and up to date list of Research, Donations and Reparations Organizations can be found here www.susannabarkataki.com/ reparationsorganizations

We are committed to support embracing yoga's roots and communities impacted by systemic oppression and injustice as we work to create equity.

HUMANITARIAN AID IN INDIA

National Campaign on Dalit Human Rights - http://www.ncdhr.org.in/
Action Aid India—https://www.actionaidindia.org/
Maitri India—https://maitriindia.org/
Sarvodaya—Service-Based Social Change https://www.sarvodaya.org/

YOGA-BASED SERVICE/SCHOOLS IN INDIA

Manav Sadhna http://www.manavsadhna.org/
Kushi Yoga Academy—https://www.khushi.org.in/

CRAFT/ART

Chhoti Si Asha—https://www.chhotisiasha.org/;
One can support their work through: www.rhope.org
Manzil—http://www.manzil.in/

U.S.- BASED ORGANIZATIONS

South Asian Mental Health Organization—https://samhin.org/
Equality Labs - www.equalitylabs.org
SAALT—(South Asian Americans Leading Together)—http://saalt.org/
SATRANG—Serving South Asian LGBTQ—http://satrang.org/
Sakhi For South Asian Women—http://www.sakhi.org/
The Sikh Coalition—https://www.sikhcoalition.org/
South Asian Women's Creative Collective—http://www.sawcc.org/

BLACK AND INDIGENOUS ORGANIZATIONS

Black Lives Matter - Global Network is a chapter-based, member-led organization whose mission is to build local power and to intervene in violence inflicted on Black communities by the state and vigilantes.

Dignity and Power Now - Abolitionist organization working to end incarceration and support communities with arts and wellness.

Minnesota Freedom Fund - Abolitionist organization working to free incarcerated folks of color and end the criminal injustice system.

Sistersong- strengthens and amplifies the collective voices of indigenous women and women of color to achieve reproductive justice by eradicating reproductive oppression and securing human rights.

Global Fund For Women - Global organization that protects the rights of women, especially women of color, worldwide.

Indigenous World - Global Human Rights organization dedicated to preserving rights of Indigenous people worldwide.

The First Nations COVID Emergency Fund - Funding for Indigenous communities hardest hit by health crises.

MODIFIABLE LETTER TO NON-REPRESENTATIONAL YOGA EVENT, TRAINING, SUMMIT, WORKSHOP, FESTIVAL

Hello,

Your [*Insert Event Here*] looks very interesting. I'm thinking of coming and participating and I'd like to know more.

As far as I understand it, yoga is a tradition from India, created, founded and professionalized by Brown and Black people for thousands of years and also still currently. I have questions about how your event lineup looks like it does.

I'm curious to know how many South Asian yogis and other yogis of color you asked to end up with this imbalanced representation?

Please contact me if you need suggestions of yoga leaders.

I do hope you are willing to engage in this conversation in the spirit of yoga—integrity, honesty, *ahimsa* (accountability) and *satya* (truth-telling). I look forward to hearing your thoughts.

Thank you.
Sincerely,
[Your Name]
Contact information

SUSTAINABLE UNITY WITH YOGA

Devotion is that which generates knowledge... knowledge is that which fashions freedom."

– Tulsidas

WE HAVE TRAVELED TOGETHER ON THIS JOURNEY, AIMING TO RESTORE the authenticity and diversity yoga deserves while deepening our own practice.

Wherever you and I are, there is universal connection available to us right here and now.

Though we are separate, we are also connected. We share a deep love and appreciation for a practice that reminds us every moment to find unity and connection to one another.

I'm sitting on my sofa, wondering how to finish this book, when an image flashes clearly to mind. I remember a moment when I was called from another sofa to an outer journey. I was living in the South of India for a while and left my cousin's home in Bangalore, India to take pilgrimage to visit the caves of *Ellora* in a remote region of *Maharashtra*, India. I was called to *Ellora* for a deeply personal reason, beyond just seeing a UNESCO World Heritage site built from the 5th - 10th century. I know our ancestors have much to share and I wanted to see what unity might just look like with my own eyes.

Upon arriving at the foot of the golden basalt mountains, I sucked in my breath with awe. In front of me rose living testament to thousands of years of worship, art, faith, compassion and unity in diversity, side by side.

I took in towering intricate carvings, created over hundreds of centuries, hollowed out of stone. To the left, a huge *Jain* cave. To the center, a large *Hindu* cave sculpture. To the right an elaborate Buddhist temple. For hundreds of years, spiritual practitioners, artists, craftspeople, families lived side by side, practicing different versions of the divine, without battle or strife. This is what beauty in diversity, harmony and unity can feel like.

Yoga today, like each of us, has so much potential. It means unity. But today, it is anything but this. Watered down yoga will not serve us now.

Though yoga means *yuj*, unity, joining or yoking, it also means harmony.

Harmony happens when there is no separation.

We have before us a vehicle of yogic consciousness to be shared with all beings. We can build bridges, and even caves, to dissolve separations within and without with our practice.

Our yoga integrity check-in invites us to show up to yoga so fully and completely that we are completely all in. We are so dedicated to yoga that we no longer experience separation between thought and desire, between self and other.

We can explore together as modern-day inquirers, seekers, yogis, purpose finders, coaches, adventurers, mystics, spiritual practitioners, and people who know there is more to the story. Together, we can lean back on authentic yoga culture as a vessel for shaping change now.

Success with Embracing Yoga's Roots comes to life when we create a world where yoga is unity and excludes no one. We have the opportunity to practice for honoring ourselves, each other, and living a global practice for sustainability and care.

Can you join in proclaiming and living that?

Yoga is here for us to cultivate power and transcend our very limitations, personally, culturally and socially. Not to create more separation but as a way to connect, dissolving separation within and without.

We can rely on yoga itself. We can lean back while practicing forward to a future that makes separation an outdated practice of the past. This is possible for you and I, in our lifetimes. It is a message and a practice that is needed more than ever.

It is this experience of global empathy and unity in diversity I hope you carry with you from this book. Though we may have different experiences and different ways of doing this work, we share a deep love of yoga and can each do our part to embrace yoga's roots. By exploring, practicing and living in this way, we create a sustainable future of care and true union that is of great contribution to ourselves, our families, students and communities as well as to the legacy of yoga.

ABOUT THE AUTHOR

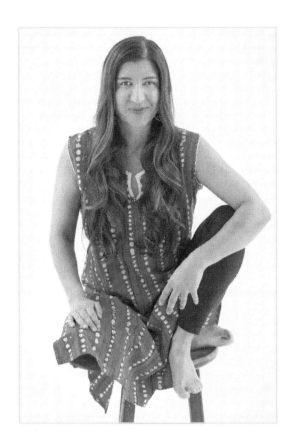

I HAVE BEEN ON A JOURNEY TO DISCOVERING UNITY MY WHOLE LIFE, perhaps because I felt so alone and separate. I studied yoga and *Ayurveda* as a pathway to reclaiming a heritage that had been taken from me.

As a mixed Indian and British-born child living in the U.S., my life has been a dance between reconciling past strengths, challenges and injustices in order to survive and thrive today.

Now, I am a student of yoga first and foremost. I am honored to teach, speak and write for an international audience. To bring critical thinking, disruption and ancient practices of unity where they are needed most.

But it certainly didn't start this way. My early years were a mess of painful alienation. Escaping racial violence against us, my family immigrated to the

U.S. from England when I was 5. Looking for a place accepting of diversity, they chose L.A. Unfortunately, we moved to a very racist part of the San Fernando Valley.

Part of why I didn't fit in was because I was the only Brown girl on the block and one of three Brown girls in my class. That made a difference that my schoolmates didn't let me forget.

I was tormented for my Brown skin. There were three 7-year-old white boys on the corner of my street, and I would spend many waking hours ignoring the taunts of "Darkie," "You smell" and "Go back to where you came from, terrorist." Dodging and weaving through them as I tried to go about my day was painful.

But the disconnect wasn't just the external. There was a process of reconciling happening within me that I couldn't articulate or explain. I was always asking why, why, why? I wanted to know the depth and purpose behind things and the greater meaning to suffering, to joy, to life all around us.

I devoted my life to the practice and study of yoga because I had no other choice. If I hadn't found a way to unify the separation within and around me, I wouldn't have survived. My whole growth path has been a practice of yoga, of unity, and I have seen it bring so much healing.

Through yoga I was able to transform from an angry, anxious and alienated girl to a thoughtful, clear, focused and positive young woman. I grew from the painfully shy person who ran out of the room at the mention of giving a speech into someone who taught more than 3,500 students in World, U.S. History and Literature over 16 years, and who now teaches large groups and presents on international stages.

Through yoga, I have been able to reconnect with my roots and find joy in who I am and where I come from, to transform self-hate and internalized oppression to self-care and even self-love. It is yoga that enables me to have compassion for my tormentors and even enemies. Yoga that lets me turn from caring for myself only to caring for others. Through yoga I began to understand the politics and the spirituality of nonviolent social change.

Yoga has fueled my lifelong pursuit of *seva*—of service for social justice.

Yoga gives me the tools to create transformation in many communities I've lived in by applying yoga in action with nonviolent tools.

I rely on the theoretical, practical and spiritual work of those who have come before, such as the many nonviolent civil resisters to colonization, Vinoba Bhave, A.T. Ariaratne, Satish Kumar, S.N. Goenka, B. R. Ambedkar, Frantz Fanon, Thich Nhat Hanh, Vandana Shiva, as well as many others.

This book is a mirror of my own journey of yoga. A process of reconciliation, to the British and Indian parts of myself, the colonizer and colonized, the yogi and activist, healer and healing. Sharing self-acceptance, integrity and unity.

This book is a testament to what is possible with the power of a life lived in yoga.

This book is also a love letter to you, a wish that you may cease to experience or create separation. That you may heal through reflection again and again, and continue to find the depth of practice and unity that the ancients lived and showed us is possible so that we may share it with future generations.

PRAISE FOR

SUSANNA BARKATAKI,
TEACHER & EQUITY CONSULTANT

"Susanna Barkataki elevates our understanding of yoga. It is beyond time to wake up and shift the paradigm that is pervading yoga today and honor the teachings with integrity, taking responsibility for how we practice and teach."

—TRACEE STANLEY,
FOUNDER, SANKALPA SHAKTI YOGA SCHOOL AND CO-FOUNDER, EMPOWERED WISDOM YOGA NIDRA TRAINING SCHOOL

"I highly recommend her teachings as a way to educate and build awareness of cultural erasure and cultural appropriation of yoga in the West."

—ANUSHA WIJEYAKUMAR,
FOUNDER WOC AND WELLNESS

"As I reflect on all I learned in our class, I feel a deep sense of *gratitude*. Serendipitous. This path that led me into your space."

—KRISTEN HANNA

"There are few opportunities where we are given the gift to answer the call of ancestors to carry their work for humanity forward into the next generation. Susanna has answered the call and this work is now our gift."

—JASMINE HINES,
PRINCIPAL CONSULTANT, THE INSPOWER AGENCY

"Susanna you changed my life! Before taking part in your course I felt like giving up yoga altogether! I was so frustrated and hurt by the current yoga scene and I felt like I was the only one who felt that way…then I joined and I was just in awe of all this knowledge and of course by the union I felt!"

—JULIA FELBAR,
YOGA PRACTITIONER

"Her energy is amazing. And her street cred is unarguable. This course will provide you with a roadmap to true yoga and deepen whatever it is you want to spend your time and life doing."

—AMBER LEINO,
YOGA TEACHER TRAINER

"There is something about the questions you pose and the way you pose them. It touches a place of deep knowing in me—knowing that things are off, knowing that I have work to do, and also knowing that you support that work and that we can actually make changes for the better."

—LIZ BUCAR

"Susanna is an amazing teacher and yogi. It's easy to learn and stay motivated when you have such a wonderful and enthusiastic teacher."

—MELANIE LEWIS,
ACTRESS

"Susanna is an amazing spiritual guide and I feel blessed beyond words to have experienced the joy of studying with her. After studying with Susanna, I feel more at peace with myself and my place in the world."

—BARBARA MEYER,
RYT 500

"THIS is what the Western yoga world has been missing. Susanna's intersectional view point is an integral piece that can support instructors and practitioners in holding themselves accountable to being in right relationship with this ancient practice."

—LUNA GRACE ISBELL LOVE,
WOMAN OF DEVOTION, MENTOR

"I have been practicing Yoga for over 16 years and leading group as well as private sessions for 6. I wanted my next training to go beyond physical practice. I have been inspired to follow my soul vision and truly walk my higher path. This has been one of the most transforming

and healing experiences of my life. I have deep gratitude for Susanna and am eternally thankful for her guidance."

—LISA STARR,
RYT 500

"This is a long-awaited and rare opportunity to learn from a South Asian yoga teacher and scholar. May the information in this book be a reminder of the infinite possibilities to collectively heal and transform simply by choosing to prioritize inclusion and restoration."

—SARA CLARK,
MINDFULNESS COACH &
EYT 500-HOUR CERTIFIED
YOGA TEACHER

"The course curriculum focuses on yoga's roots and honors its cultural significance. I am so grateful for learning to create a community of inclusivity and cultivating the yogic lifestyle."

—SUSANA CASTRO,
RYT 500

"Your course changed the way I see myself and the world."

—KATHRYN FEQUETTE

LEARN, CONNECT, CONTINUE TO DO THIS WORK

As a companion to take the work of this book deeper into your life and practice, Susanna has created a quick and powerful 4-part Embrace Yoga's Roots Online Course for you as a complement to the book.

The course offers tools, meditations and specific, easy-to-understand steps to deepen an honoring personal practice with action steps that take you into the heart of what yoga has to offer.

Join Susanna to take this work further in the Embrace Yoga Online Course. Deepen Your Practice, Avoid Appropriation, Embrace Yoga's Roots and Embody Yoga Leadership.

**LEARN to practice and teach to embrace yoga's roots
and get a bundle of free resources to Embrace Yoga:**
www.embraceyogaresources.com

More learning opportunities:
Free masterclass on how to confidently start and end your
yoga class without offending without intention at
www.namastemasterclass.com.

Watch/listen to interviews with 40+ experts by Susanna
Barkataki at www.honordontappropriateyoga.com.

CONNECT

Follow Susanna's Insta-gations and Blogs on
Instagram and Her Site

www.instagram.com/susannabarkataki
www.susannabarkataki.com

CONTINUE

**Train with Susanna in her Embody
Yoga's Roots Yoga Teacher Trainings 200/300/500**
www.ignitebewell.com

**Embrace Yoga's Roots Workshops in your
YTTs, studios and schools**
To book Susanna write: booking@ignitebewell.com

ORGANIZATIONAL SUPPORT

Susanna Barkataki offers transformational workshops and
trainings to help organizations shift culture to be inclusive,
mindful and diverse.
For inquires about speaking, workshops and trainings
write:
booking@ignitebewell.com.

OPPORTUNITIES FOR YOU AND YOUR ORGANIZATION

ARE YOU RUNNING A YOGA STUDIO, WELLNESS CENTER, NONPROFIT OR YTT?

Do you want your staff educated about equity, diversity, inclusion, cultural appropriation and grounded in authentic yoga knowledge?

Do your company's mission, strategies and practices include efforts to support diversity and inclusion through education?

How are you cultivating a culture of mindfulness and health in your organization, and are yoga and meditation a part of that?

Whether you operate in the yoga culture landscape or not, if you want to ensure your organization honors yoga's roots while complying with inclusion and diversity requirements, Susanna Barkataki and IGNITE Yoga and Wellness Institute have options to support your efforts through our special offers:

- **Bulk sales** discounts for both the paperback and eBook versions of *Embrace Yoga's Roots*, starting with as few as 10 books.

- **Co-branding** for your special bulk purchase. We can create a custom version of *Embrace Yoga's Roots*, co-branding with your organization, including your logo on the front cover and a page inside devoted to your organization.

- **Online Support** delivering Susanna's companion **Embrace Yoga's Roots Online Course** to the next-level yoga leader who wants to deepen their practice while respecting rather than appropriating.

Designed as the companion to *Embrace Yoga's Roots*, we'll help you share this groundbreaking content at a discounted price, even creating a custom bundle of the book and the course, for your YTT or as a continuing education course for your students.

- **Consulting, Speaking, Keynotes, Training and YTTs** with Susanna in your Yoga Teacher Training program, board meetings, company events or conference. She will deliver an event designed to reach your team with great skill, compassion and humor grounded in knowledge, resources and tools to implement inclusion, equity, diversity and unity.

Explore these options with Susanna and be on the leading edge of this paradigm shift—where we learn to honor traditions, apply them in our modern world and deepen our connections to each other with respect, cultural competence and unity.

FOR MORE INFORMATION, CONTACT:
booking@ignitebewell.com

ACKNOWLEDGMENTS

To the devoted practitioners and teachers of yoga *dharma* across time and space. I am forever in your awe and debt. To my teachers Shankaracharya, Thich Nhat Hanh, Caitriona Reed, Michelle Benzamin-Miki, Eisha Mason, Dr. Tara Sethia, Arundhati Roy, A.T. Ariaratne, Satish Kumar, S.N. Goenka, B. R. Ambedkar, Vandana Shiva, as well as many others who have taught me—I am deeply grateful. Grateful beyond words and even beyond thought.

Thank you, Eran James. "I'd always bet on anything she does" are the most amazing words any partner can hear. To Kailash James for believing in yourself, the power of books, reading and imagination. Starting your **Make Book Factory** during my writing process is the biggest vote of confidence that any mom could receive. I'll certainly bet on anything you do and I look forward to publishing our shared work *The Adventures of Monk and Nun* soon!

To the community of the diasporas—you know who you are and I have your back always. You've helped me become who I am.

To Cathy and Shan Barkataki and all my family, thank you for being there. Supporting and shaping me into who I am. I love you.

My beloved and wise teachers and coaches Sonali Fiske, Luna Love, Shereen Sun, who kept me unblocked, inspired and the words flowing.

For my early readers Aditi Desai, Jacoby Ballard, Constanza Eliana Chinea, Kelsey Rust and Eran James for your time and thought in every edit. Thank you.

To my dear friends and confidants Neelam Pathikonda, Ariane White, Xochitl Ashe, Samantha Santiago and the wide and deep Embrace Yoga community. To the South Asian, Indian, Desi, Black, Brown BIPOC community. We are waking up. We are here. It's time we take our rightful place and I'm so honored to do this work alongside you. You are amazing.

Thank you for your expertise, wise advice, editing and belief in the cause Michelle Vandepas, Kelly Madrone and Michelle Morgan. Thank you to Melinda Martin and Minhajul Islam for your patient formatting genius. Thank you Amber DeDerick for your inspired detailed indexing. Thank you to Camille Truman for everything. You bring this work alive with knowledge, design, passion and care.

Thank you to Catarina Andrade, Tiwanna Shipp and Emily Jackson for your every single effort. You made so much more possible.

To all of my students. Past, present and future. I would not be without you. To you I bow with unending gratitude and reverence.

To everyone who has been touched by and cares about yoga. To embodying it now and preserving it for the future. This is for us. This is it.

GLOSSARY

This glossary gives definitions of working terms used in the book. It is not meant to be exhaustive but to define concepts and terms used in this context. Use this as a jumping-off point to learn more. One place to start is to search the index to look up the terms used to gain more understanding of these terms in context.

Ābhyanga Ayurvedic practice of self-care and massage with warmed oil.

Abhyāsa Consistent effort. Often paired with the letting go of 3.

Accessibility Refers to the design of products, devices, services or environments for people who experience disabilities.

Accomplice Someone who uses their privilege to address and dismantle systems of oppression.

Advaita Vedanta Nondual form of yoga and Hinduism. Belief in interconnection, oneness and unity of all things.

Āhimsa Non-harm, kindness.

Ally Someone who advocates for and supports members of a community other than their own. Reaching across differences to achieve mutual goals.

Ambedkar, B.R. A socialist, activist and social reformer who inspired many Dalits to convert to Buddhism to disrupt caste oppression.

Angulimala Historic figure who was known to harm many people but then met the Buddha and converted to Buddhism and became a monk.

Anuloma Viloma Otherwise known as alternate nostril breathing; a calming breathing technique where one breathes in and out through one nostril and then the other.

Aparigraha Letting go, nonattachment.

Āsana Seat, posture. The physical practice of yoga postures.

Ashoka Emperor who wanted to share this path of non-violence with the world.

Asteya Non-stealing, generosity.

Atman The divine, the Self.

Aum Sacred sound.

Āyurveda A system of healing and wellness that originated in India. This ancient Indian science of wellbeing comes from *ayuh* meaning "life" or "longevity" and *veda* meaning "study of."

Bandhas Energy locks or seals in the body.

Bhagavad Gita 700-Verse Sanskrit scripture and a foundational text of yogic knowledge and wisdom.

Bhajans Spiritual songs of devotion.

Bhakti School of yoga that focuses on devotion.

Bias Preference for or against something; likes or dislikes.

Bindu Drop or point.

Bindi Spiritual adornment, often a red or other colored dot on the forehead to signify various spiritual meanings.

BIPOC Black Indigenous People of Color

Bodhisattva A being who has committed to a spiritual path of ending suffering for all beings, usually in Buddhism.

Brahmacharya Awareness of the divine; constraint of energy.

Chakra Wheel. Energy center in the body.

Chandogya Upanishad One of the oldest sacred texts of the *Sama Veda*.

Colonialism System of oppression fulfilled by controlling a country, occupying it, settling it and exploiting its natural resources, cultural and indigenous wealth.

Cultural Appropriation Taking something from a culture that is not one's own. Involves privilege and a power imbalance plus harm to the source culture. The harm can be of disrespect and also of material, cultural, financial, economic, social and spiritual harm.

Decolonization Working to restore the original ownership of the land and resources from those of whom they have been taken or stolen. Also used to refer to a process of undoing the mindset of being colonized.

Dehumanize To make a person seem less human in order to justify mistreatment.

Desi Diasporic Indians who live outside India.

Dharana Mindfulness and focus.

Dharma Purpose, law, divine order.

Dhyana Meditation.

Discrimination The unjust treatment and acting-out of prejudice in a way that harms a person or group based on identity, such as race, class, gender identity, sexual expression, etc.

Diversity Respecting, including and celebrating differences. These can be along the dimensions of race, ethnicity, gender, sexual orientation, socio-economic status, age, physical abilities, religious beliefs, political beliefs or other identifying factors.

Diya Candle, light.

Dosha A colloquial term often used in *Ayurveda* to refer to a unique mind-body-spirit type in *Ayurveda*. The *doshas* are made up of the five elements and are called *vata*, *pitta* and *kapha*.

Drishti Focus and steadiness of the gaze.

East Asians People who are from China, Korea, Japan, Taiwan, Tibet or Mongolia.

Epistemology The study of what we know and how we know it.

Equity Giving everyone what they need to be successful, taking into account the vast diversity of structural privilege, power and oppression, and life experience. Equity identifies and strives to eliminate blocks that have prevented some groups or people from participating fully.

Fakir A spiritual renunciate, usually in a Sufi Muslim context.

Glamorization A practice of cultural appropriation involving taking cultural practices out of context and putting them on for the purpose of looking exotic or cool.

Guru A respected or esteemed teacher, usually one who holds a position in a teaching lineage.

Guru-parampara Guru lineage passed from teacher to student.

Gurukul The traditional model of teaching given by a guru in very small groups or one to one.

Healing Justice A movement led by BIPOC that acknowledges the healing tools and power of our ancestors and acknowledges that our illnesses or maladies are not individual events but are socially created, so healing and the creation of wellness must take into account justice.

Heteronormativity A prejudiced belief, based on the gender binary, that heterosexuality is the typical or normal orientation.

Inclusion An intention or policy of including people who might otherwise be excluded or marginalized, such as those who are handicapped or learning-disabled, or racial and sexual minorities.

Indigenous Native to a place, people or practice.

Institutional Oppression Arrangement of a society used to benefit one group at the expense of another through the use of language, media, education, religion, economics, etc.

Internalized Oppression The result and the process by which an oppressed person comes to believe, accept or live out the inaccurate stereotypes and misinformation about their group.

Intersectionality An important conceptual term coined by Kimberlé Crenshaw, it refers to how categories like race, class, gender, sexuality and ability are interconnected and work together to affect our individual and collective experiences. The concept also explains how these categories correlate to different, yet connected, systems of oppression, power and privilege.

Ishvara Pranidhana Devotion to the divine and study of sacred texts.

Japa mantra Repetition of sacred sound intended to calm the mind.

Jnana yoga School of yoga that focuses on study and knowledge.

Kapha is conceived of the elements earth and water and correlates to the quality of heaviness and the emotions of depression and steadiness.

Karma yoga School of yoga that focuses on action.

Karma Action, taking personal responsibility.

Kirtan Spiritual songs of devotion often sung in a call-and-response style.

Lineage From where a student has learned their yogic knowledge.

Mahabharata An epic poem of conflict.

Malas Prayer beads.

Mandir Temple.

Mantra Sacred sound.

Metaphysics The study of what is real.

Metta Loving kindness.

Microaggressions Everyday actions, slights, indignities, put-downs and insults that target populations (minorities, women, LGBTQ+ people) experience in their day-to-day lives. Microaggressions are part of a system of inequity and add up for those who are the targets of them.

Mudra Sacred gesture.

Nalanda A large monastery and place of study and learning with scholars from many lineages, primarily in the Buddhist tradition.

Namaste A Sanskrit sacred greeting for elders.

Neo-Colonial Colonization has not ended; it has continued but changed forms. Neo-colonial describes modern methods of colonialism, which largely involve capitalism, globalism and cultural imperialism.

Niyama Inner yogic codes.

Ontology The study of how we know what we know.

Oppression Political, economic, social, cultural putting-down of people, groups or individuals.

Orientalism Defined by Edward Said, describes often oversexualized, infantilized, exotic and patronizing descriptions of people of the East.

Orientalization To give Asian stereotypes or qualities to things or people that are not Asian.

Patanjali 2nd/3rd-century sage who is credited with codifying and writing the *Yoga Sutras.*

Pitta Doshic quality of fire, composed of air and water elements, corresponds to emotions of anger and clarity.

POC People of Color.

Post-Colonial The belief that colonization has ended.

Power Over External power to control, dominate or enact one's will over another.

Power The ability to affect one's will on the world and create change.

Power With Power used for uplifting, supporting or helping another person or group.

Power Within Internal power. This is a power that cannot be given or taken away.

Prakriti Our unique, distinctive constitution or mind-body-spirit type.

Pranayama Breath and life force.

Prejudice A pre-judgment about someone or something based on assumptions.

Privilege Unearned advantages.

Race Human beings classified as a more or less distinct group because of shared physical traits, such as skin color.

Racism (Discrimination + power) Any attitude, action or practice backed up by institutional power that harms people because they belong to a particular racial group; a system of social, economic, political or other advantage/privilege bestowed on people who possess certain physical trait(s).

Raja Kingly yoga, or complete yoga.

Renunciate One who gives up the pleasures of the world in order to focus on spiritual growth and attainment.

Reparations Atoning for what has been stolen and returning many of the benefits, rights and profits of a culture's inheritance to its creators and culture.

Resource Anything that creates a sense of internal safety, enabling us to explore, unpack and make sense of a past experience.

Rishi Vedic term for a sage or someone who is enlightened.

Samadhi Bliss, liberation.

Samyama The combined practice of *dharana* (mindfulness), *dhyana* (concentration) and *samadhi* (bliss), otherwise known as insight states accessible during meditation.

Sankalpa Deep, heartfelt, soul-level intention.

Santosha Joy.

Sanyasi A renunciate who casts aside worldly concerns of money, stature or comfort in pursuit of spiritual aims, usually in yogic tradition.

Satya Truth.

Satyagraha Truth force.

Saucha Keeping one's mind and body pure and clean.

Seva Service and devotion.

Sevagram Ashram *Ashram* of many faiths and practitioners established by Mahatma Gandhi in Wardha, India.

Shakti Power.

Shantideva Buddhist monk and scholar at Nālandā University in India around 700 C.E.

Shavasana Yogic rest.

Shimla Hill station in Northern India and beautiful honeymoon and tourist destination spot.

Siddhartha Gautama Enlightened person and teacher from 2nd century C.E. known as the *Buddha*.

Sikh People associated with Sikhism, a monotheistic religion developed in the 15th century C.E.

South Asian People who are from Afghanistan, Pakistan, India, Bangladesh, Nepal, Bhutan, Sri Lanka or Maldives.

Southeast Asians Come from countries that are south of China, east of India. This includes eleven countries: Thailand, Vietnam, Malaysia, Singapore, the Philippines, Laos, Indonesia, Brunei, Burma (Myanmar), Cambodia and East Timor.

Spiritual Lineage Acknowledgment Making an effort to name and acknowledge the spiritual roots of the practice of yoga in India as well as naming one's teachers.

***Sri Adi Shankaracharya* (also *Adi Shankara*)** An Indian teacher and saint from the 8th century C.E. who helped revive *advaita vedanta* and spread yogic teachings through a system of monasteries.

Stereotype A belief about a group that doesn't take individual differences into account.

Sterilization A form of cultural appropriation that occurs when one sanitizes the practice by taking the cultural elements out of yoga to make it more palatable to the dominant culture.

Svadhyaya Self-inquiry.

Swadesh Self-rule.

Swami Spiritual practitioner or teacher.

Swaraj Self-rule, independence. Can be used personally or politically.

Systemic Oppression The political, economic, social, cultural putting-down of people, groups or individuals.

Tai Chi An East Asian martial art.

Tapas Yogic discipline and austerity practice.

Tokenizing Treating a member of a group as if they are a representative of the whole group.

Trauma Anything overwhelming that impacts the nervous system in a way in which we are unable to cope or respond and causes fragmentation in mind-body-spirit.

Upanishad Sitting at the feet of a sage or teacher. Sacred texts from the Vedic tradition.

Using Privilege Leveraging privilege to uplift others.

Vata Dosha is elements air and space, associated with movement and correlates with the emotions of creativity and anxiety.

Veda Ancient Sanskrit texts.

Vichara Self-inquiry.

Viveka Discernment.

Warda Village in central India where Gandhi set up *Sevagram Ashram* and nonviolent activists live and work to this day.

White People whose origins come from Europe.

White Centering Holding white experience, white feelings, white stories and narratives as the center of all experiences. Discrediting, ignoring or devaluing perspectives from BIPOC. Unintentionally or intentionally treating Black Indigenous people of color as less-than and excluding or erasing them, their feelings, views, stories, experiences or perspectives.

White Supremacists White nationalism. A belief that is pro-white and explicitly anti-black or anti-people-of-color.

White Supremacy A system of power that privileges white people and posits that white people are fundamentally superior, better, more intelligent than other people. The belief that white people are superior to all other races and that they should therefore hold the highest positions in society and dominate all other races.

WOC Women of Color.

Yama Yoga ethics.

Yamas **and** *Niyamas* The **yamas** and **niyamas** are ethical foundations of yoga. They represent a yogic vision for a global yoga practice, lifestyle and ethic.

Yoga A spiritual practice that originated in South Asia. The Sanskrit word *yoga* describes both a state of the union, oneness or connection in consciousness and experience as well as the techniques, philosophies, practices and lifestyles that bring one to such a state. The development, codification and practice aimed at engendering oneness we understand as yoga has been practiced, cultivated and explored over time, particularly on the Indian subcontinent, for thousands of years. Today, what we understand as yoga explores this interconnected state of consciousness, along with the development of physical health, emotional regulation and wellbeing.

Yogashastra A book of knowledge or teaching about yoga.

Yoga Nidra Yogic relaxation and rest.

Yoga Sadhana Practice, the deepening of these many and varied practices.

REFERENCES

Ackerman, Courtney. (2018). "What is Neuroplasticity? A Psychologist Explains." https://positivepsychology.com/neuroplasticity/ (Accessed 6/10/19).

Adams, M., L. A. Bell, and P. Griffin, eds. (2007). *Teaching for Diversity and Social Justice: A Sourcebook*, 2nd ed. New York: Routledge.

Adichi Chimamanda. (2017). "The Danger of a Single Story." TED Talk. https://www.youtube.com/watch?v=D9Ihs241zeg

Ali, Zahra. *Ignite Yoga Teacher Training*, Discussion, Sept 1, 2019.

Andre, Christof. (2019). "Proper Breathing Brings Better Health." *Scientific American*. https://www.scientificamerican.com/article/proper-breathing-brings-better-health/ (Accessed 1/17/2019).

Anonymous (2002). Ignite!—An Anti-Racist Toolkit.

Barkataki, Susanna. (2015). "The Paradise We are Missing with Self Care." https://www.huffpost.com/entry/the-paradise-we-are-missi_b_8137410

Barkataki, Susanna. (2019). "From Harm to Respect." *Yoga Girl Blog*. https://www.yogagirl.com/read/yoga/5d0xi27wt2CwOEm28MWW0e

Basavaraddi, Dr. Ishwar V. (2015) "Yoga: Its Origin, History and Development."

Brown, Adrienne Maree. (2017). *Emergent Strategy*. Chico, California: AK Press.

Chimamanda, A. (2017). "The Dangers of a Single Narrative." Ted Talk.

Clemens, C. (2017). *Ally or Accomplice? The Language of Activism*. https://www.tolerance.org/magazine/ally-or-accomplice-the-language-of-activism (Accessed 6/15/19).

CNBC. (2018). "Lululemon Shares Soar as Earnings top Expectations." https://www.cnbc.com/2018/08/30/lululemon-earnings-q2-2018.html

Cook, Jubilee & Rain, Karen. How to Respond to Sexual Abuse Within a Yoga or Spiritual Community. Yoga International. 2020. https://yogainternational.com/article/view/how-to-respond-to-sexual-abuse-within-a-yoga-or-spiritual-community

Crenshaw, Kimberlé. (1989). Demarginalizing the Intersection of Race and Sex: A Black Feminist Critique of Antidiscrimination Doctrine, Feminist Theory and Antiracist Politics. *University of Chicago Legal Forum*, Volume 1989, Article 8.

Crenshaw, Kimberlé. (2017). Kimberlé Crenshaw on Intersectionality, More than Two Decades Later, *Columbia Law Review*. https://www.law.columbia.edu/pt-br/news/2017/06/kimberle-crenshaw-intersectionality

Crosby, Kim. *Allyship, Intersectionality, and Anti-Oppression.* http://prezi.com/nesv_ekel126/allyship-intersectionality-anti-oppression/

Cull, Ian, Hancock, Robert L. A. McKeown, Stephanie, Pidgeon, Michelle, and Vedan, Adrienne. *Decolonization and Indigenization.* https://opentextbc.ca/indigenizationfrontlineworkers/chapter/decolonization-and-indigenization/ (Accessed 1/20/20).

Dalai Lama, XIV; Padmakara Translation Group. (1994). *A Flash of Lightning in the Dark of Night: Guide to the Bodhisattva's Way of Life,* 1st ed. Boston: Shambhala.

Descartes, Renee. (November 19, 2010). *Meditations on First Philosophy.* Gearhart, Oregon: Watchmaker Publishing (first published 1641).

Deshpande, Rina. (2019). "What's the Difference Between Cultural Appropriation and Cultural Appreciation?" *Yoga Journal.*

Diaz, R. (2017). "Challenging the 'White Ally' Model: To Defeat Racism, We All Need to Dismantle Racial Capitalism." http://inthesetimes.com/article/20459/white-ally-racism-charlottesville-capitalism (Accessed 6/23/19).

Doran, Louiza, and Lebron, T. (2019). *That's Not How That Works,* Episode 43 https://www.stitcher.com/podcast/trudi-lebron/hey-auntie/e/59405027?autoplay=true

EGangotri, Mrigendra Samhita Vivritti Bhatta Narayan. (1999). Alm 9 Shlf 2 Devanagari Tantra. https://archive.org/details/MrigendraSamhitaVivrittiBhattaNarayan1999Alm9Shlf2Devanagari Tantra/page/n1 (Accessed 9/10/19).

Eisler, Riane. (2007). *The Real Wealth of Nations: Creating a Caring Economics.* Oakland, California: Berrett-Koehler Publishers.

Emerson, Dave. (2015). *Trauma-Sensitive Yoga in Therapy: Bringing the Body into Treatment,* 1st ed. New York: W. W. Norton & Company.

Fabello, Melissa A. (2015). *Self-Care 101: What It is and Where to Start.* https://everydayfeminism.com/2015/02/self-care-101/ (Accessed 7/17/19).

Gandhi, Mohandas, K. (1983). *Mohandas K. Gandhi, Autobiography: The Story of My Experiments with Truth.* New York: Dover Publications.

Gandhi, Shreena and Wolff, Lillie. (2017). "Yoga and the Roots of Cultural Appropriation." Kalamazoo College. https://www.kzoo.edu/praxis/yoga/ (Accessed 12/19/19).

Gehl, Lynn. "Bill of Responsibilities." http://www.lynngehl.com/my-ally-bill-of-responsibilities.html (Accessed 11/10/19).

Goodman, D. (2001). *Promoting diversity and social justice: Educating people from privileged groups.* Thousand Oaks, CA: Sage.

Heyman, Jivana. (2018). *Accessible Yoga.* Boston: Shambhala.

Hickel, Jason. Britain Stole 45 Trillion from India. (2018) https://www.aljazeera.com/indepth/opinion/britain-stole-45-trillion-india-181206124830851.html (Accessed 1/20/20).

hooks, bell. (2015). *Understanding Patriarchy.* https://imaginenoborders.org/pdf/zines/UnderstandingPatriarchy.pdf (Accessed 1/10/20).

hooks, bell. (2018). *All About Love.* New York: William Morrow Paperbacks.

Indigenous Action Media. (2014). *Accomplices Not Allies: Abolishing The Ally Industrial Complex.* http://www.indigenousaction.org/accomplices-not-allies-abolishing-the-ally-industrial-complex (Accessed 1/9/20).

Iyengar. B.K.S. (1964) *Light on Yoga.* Berlin: Schocken Books.

Jackson, Catrice, M. (2017). *White Spaces Missing Faces.* Catriceology Enterprises.

Johnson, A. (2006). *Privilege, power and difference,* 2nd ed. Mountain View, CA: Mayfield.

Johnson, Allan J. (2017). *Power, Privilege and Difference.* New York: McGraw-Hill.

Johnson, Maisha. Z. (2015). "What's Wrong with Cultural Appropriation? These 9 Answers Reveal Its Harm." Everyday Feminism. https://everydayfeminism.com/2015/06/cultural-appropriation-wrong/

Johnson, Michelle Cassandra. Skill in Action. 2018.

Kamat, K.L. (2019). *The Sword of Tippu Sultan.* http://www.kamat.com/kalranga/itihas/tippu.htm (Accessed1/10/20)

Kapila, Monisha, Hines, Ericka, and Searby, Martha. (2016). "Why Diversity, Equity, and Inclusion Matter." ProInspire. https://independentsector.org/resource/why-diversity-equity-and-inclusion-matter/ (Accessed 8/18/19).

Kauanui, J. Kēhaulani. (2016). "A Structure, Not an Event: Settler Colonialism and Enduring Indigeneity." *Lateral,* 5.1.

Khouri, Hala. https://halakhouri.com/ (Accessed 1/20/20)

Kimmel, M., and A. Ferber. (2010). *Privilege: A reader,* 2nd ed. Philadelphia: Westview Press.

King Jr., Dr. Martin Luther. (1963). "Letter from Birmingham Jail." https://www.africa.upenn.edu/Articles_Gen/Letter_Birmingham.html (Accessed 1/12/20).

King, Jr. Dr. Martin Luther. (1963). "Love Your Enemies." https://kinginstitute.stanford.edu/king-papers/documents/loving-your-enemies-sermon-delivered-dexter-avenue-baptist-church (Accessed 1/15/20).

King, Sara, Dr. "Meet Dr. Sara King of Mindheart Consulting in Long Beach." Voyage LA, May 7, 2019 (Accessed 1/10/20).

Kivel, P. (2002). *Uprooting racism: How white people can work for racial justice.* Gabriola Island, British Columbia, Canada: New Society Press.

Kivel, P. (2016). *Guidelines for White Allies.* http://www.racialequitytools. org/resourcefiles/kivel3.pdf (Accessed 7/21/19).

Klein, Melanie C. and Heagberg, Kat (2020). "*Embodied Resilience through Yoga: 30 Mindful Essays About Finding Empowerment After Addiction, Trauma, Grief, and Loss.*" with Jan Adams (Author), Nicole Lang (Author), Kathryn Ashworth (Author), Colin Hall (Author), Jill Weiss Ippolito (Author), Toni Willis (Author), David Holzer (Author), Jennifer Kreatsoulas PhD (Author), Mary Higgs (Author), Sarah Garden (Author), Amanda Huggins (Author), Sarah Harry (Author), Tonia Crosby (Author), Sarah Nannen (Author), Zabie Yamasaki (Author), Alli Simon (Author), Kathryn Templeton (Author), Tobias Wiggins (Author), Michael Hayes (Author), Susanna Barkataki (Author), Amber Karnes (Author), Rachel Otis (Author), Dorian Christian Baucum (Author), Niralli D'Costa (Author), Justine Mastin (Author), Sará King (Author), Kathleen Kraft (Author), Elliot Kesse (Author), Celisa Flores (Author), Antesa Jensen (Author), Sanaz Yaghmai (Author), Hala Khouri (Foreword)

Kuah, Desmond. (2016). "Timeline of British India." http://www. victorianweb.org/history/empire/india/timeline.html

Lenard, Patti, & Balint, P. (2019). *What is (the wrong of) cultural appropriation?* Ethnicities. 146879681986649. 10.1177/1468796819866498. https://www.academia.edu/40228023/ What_is_the_wrong_of_cultural_appropriation

Levine, Peter. (2006). *Trauma through a child's eyes: Awakening the ordinary miracle of healing.* Berkeley, California: North Atlantic Books.

Levine, Peter. (2007). *In an Unspoken Voice: How the Body Releases Trauma and Restores Goodness.* Berkeley, California: North Atlantic Books.

Lewis, Haley. (2018). "Indigenous People Want Brands to Stop Selling Sage and Smudge Kits." *Huffington Post.* https://www. huffingtonpost.ca/entry/indigenous-people-sage-and-smudge-kits_ca_5cd579e0e4b07bc729786e25

Lexico. (2019). *Oxford English Dictionary.* https://www.lexico.com/en/definition/colonization

Madras Courier. (2017). "How the Fakir Sanyassi Rebellion Inspired Vande Mataram." https://madrascourier.com/insight/how-the-fakir-sannyasi-rebellion-inspired-vande-mataram/

Mallinson, James and Singleton, Mark. (2017). *Roots of Yoga.* New York: Penguin Random House.

Martin, Candace. Interfaith Yoga Project. https://www.facebook.com/interfaithyogaproject/ (Accessed 1/15/20)

Nichols, Mary May. "Shankaracharya and The Four Goals of Yoga." https://digitalassets.lib.berkeley.edu/main/b20782842_C020830084.pdf (Accessed 10/12/2019).

McKenzie, Mia. (2013). No More "Allies." BGD. http://www.blackgirldangerous.org/2013/09/30/no-more-allies/

Menakem, Resmaa. (2017). *My Grandmother's Hands: Racialized Trauma and the Pathway to Mending Our Hearts and Bodies.* Central Recovery Press.

Okun, Tema, and Jones K. (2001). "White Supremacy Culture." http://www.dismantlingracism.org/uploads/4/3/5/7/43579015/whitesupcul13.pdf

Parikh, Jesal, Shah, Tejal, Yoga is Dead Podcast, Episode 1

Peterson, Eric (2017). "On Allyship and Performative Wokeness." https://medium.com/@Tawdry_Hepburn/on-allyship-and-performative-wokeness-30581808bf8b

Piepzna-Samarasinha, Leah Lakshmi. (2016). "What is Healing Justice?" https://www.advocate.com/commentary/2019/5/16/what-healing-justice

Powell, Seth. (2018). "Intro to Philosophy and History of Yoga." Online Course.

Purser, Ronald, E. (2019). *McMindfulness: How Mindfulness Became the New Capitalist Spirituality.* London: Repeater Books.

Said, Edward. *Orientalism.* (1979). New York: Vintage Books.

Tatum, Beverly Daniel. (1993). *Why are All the Black Kids Sitting Together in the Cafeteria? And Other Conversations About Race.* New York: Basic Books.

Tatum, Beverly Daniel. (2007) *Can We Talk about Race? and Other Conversations in an Era of School Resegregation.* Boston: Beacon Press.

The Anti-Oppression Network. *Allyship.* https://theantioppressionnetwork.com/allyship/ (Accessed 12/14/19).

Tuck, E. Yang, and Wayne K. (2012). "Decolonization is Not a Metaphor." *Decolonization: Indigeneity, Education, & Society* Vol.1, p. 1-40. https://www.latrobe.edu.au/staff-profiles/data/docs/fjcollins.pdf

U.S. Department of Minority Health. (2019). https://minorityhealth.hhs.gov/omh/browse.aspx?lvl=2&lvlid=26 (Accessed 12/5/19).

United States Institute for Peace. https://www.usip.org/ (Accessed 11/10/19).

Unsettling America. *Allyship & Solidarity Guidelines.* http://unsettlingamerica.wordpress.com/allyship/ (Accessed 11/10/19).

USC Calis Center. (2006). "Four Worlds of History." https://dornsife.usc.edu/calis/four-worlds-of-history/ (Accessed 9/16/19).

United States Department of Arts and Culture, (2019) https://usdac.us/nativeland (Accessed 2/15/20).

Utt, Jamie. (2013). "Things Allies Need to Know." Everyday Feminism. http://everydayfeminism.com/2013/11/things-allies-need-to-know/

Vaidya, Shaila. Dr. https://www.theyogamd.ca/

van der Kolk, Bessel. (2000). "The diagnosis and treatment of Complex PTSD." In: Yehuda R, ed. *Current Treatment of PTSD*. Washington D.C.: American Psychiatric Press.

van der Kolk, Bessel. (2015). *The Body Keeps The Score: Brain, Mind & Body.* New York: Viking.

Welwood, John. (2002). *Toward a Psychology of Awakening: Buddhism, Psychotherapy, and the Path of Personal and Spiritual Transformation,* reprint ed. Boston: Shambhala.

Wolfe, Patrick. (2006). "Settler Colonialism and the Elimination of the Native." *Journal of Genocide Research.* 8. 10.1080/14623520601056240

Yoga in America Study, (2016) IPSOS Public Affairs, Yoga Alliance and Yoga Journal https://www.yogaalliance.org/Learn/About_Yoga/2016_

Yoga_in_America_Study/Highlights (Accessed 12/20/19).

INDEX

CLOSING DEDICATION AND MEDITATION

May this work benefit all beings.
May all beings learn from, grow, respect, honor and embrace yoga.
May all beings be free of separation and the causes of separation.
May all beings reflect deeply.
May all beings act for connection.
May all beings be full of everlasting liberation.
Om Shanti Shanti Shanti
Peace within.
Peace without.
Peace in the world.
Peace, Peace, Peace.
Om Shanti Shanti Shanti

Made in the USA
Middletown, DE
16 November 2020

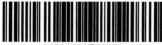

24206432R00172